Curing My Stutter

Abid

Hussain

Visit www.stammering-stuttering.com for further information

Contents

Acknowledgments

Firstly I would like to thank almighty God for guiding me in everything I do in life. I would also like to thank my mother for teaching me how to show strength in the face of adversity and for providing unrelenting love. I would like to thank my father for instilling self belief in me, being my teacher and being my dependable rock in my life.

With my deepest gratitude I wish to thank all my friends and family that have helped me with this book, you all know who you are! Most of all I would like to express my gratitude to my son Mujtaba, if it wasn't for me watching him struggle with his stutter and bringing back repressed memories of my childhood, I would not have been so motivated to write this book.

Those that know me know that I treat my family including all of my sisters as precious jewels in my life. They illuminate me, inspire me, give me strength and their light and love for me shines through regardless of the circumstances.

Introduction

Stuttering or stammering has been around for centuries. Famous stutterers include Moses, Aristotle, Napoleon and even Marilyn Monroe. Worldwide, nearly 4 percent of the population experience stuttering at some point in their lives. At any given time, about 1 percent of people stutter. This can lead to avoiding school and bullying in children.

In adults almost three quarters of people who stutter believe that they have a less chance of getting a job or a promotion because of their stutter, according to recent research. Stutterers believe that job performance is affected and they would be better at their job if they did not stutter.

Some even turn down promotions or a new job due to their stuttering.

This lack of confidence soon seeps into the social life of stutterers and can produce feelings of self hatred, anxiety and severe depression. Stutterers will commonly avoid ordering food that they find difficult to say and may limit the amount of time they spend talking to the opposite sex as a fear of humiliation may be present. In some cases stutterers have even changed their name because it contained a difficult to pronounce sound. I have stuttered myself since the age of 5 so I can truly empathise with the feelings of self hatred and anxiety.

Speaking is one of the simplest actions that fluent speaking people take for granted.

Fluent speakers would not give talking much thought or effort. For stutterers it's a different world, when we open our mouths it requires an immense amount of physical and emotional energy. When we talk three variables come into play, continuity which is talking without hesitation.

The rate or speed at which we talk and the ease of how we talk. With stutterers all three of these variables are affected.

Stuttering can involve repetitions, prolongations and external pauses with varying amounts of severity. Repetitions are common amongst stutterers as a phrase, word or syllable is repeated. An example would be "I need, to-to-to-to-to go now".

It could be a repetition of a syllable such as "I ne-ne-ne-ne-ne-need to go now." Fluent speakers can also experience mild repetition but stutterers may repeat a syllable up to 7 times.

Prolongation involves the involuntary lengthening or prolonging of vocalised speech sounds (rrrrunning, aaaapple), or non-vocalised sounds (sssseven, ffffourteen). Stuttering can also develop into a block. A block is when the first letter or syllable is very difficult to say and is effectively "blocked".

This can be very frustrating for a stutterer as they know what they want to say but the 1st syllable will not come out. What effectively happens is that the larynx (voice box) closes and stops the flow of air. Pauses are also common amongst stutterers.

There are two different types of pauses, unfilled and filled pauses. Unfilled pauses are pauses of silence during speech that is not in a common sentence structure. Filled pauses are interjections of a word with "umm", "uhh", etc. These interjections are used to ease fluency for a stutter. Each stutterer has sounds or syllables that they find difficult to say and they avoid or use interjectors to help them out. My son who also stutters uses "erm" quite a lot in between words and sometimes in the middle of a word so he may say "daaa erm daa erm dad".

Some stutterers will also have a notable twitch, excess eye movements or blinking and be unable to hold eye contact.

The life of a stutterer can go from the "good days" which are filled with relatively fluent speech and a feeling of joy and control, to the "bad days" which is when we cannot get a word out.

Now that I have explained what stuttering is and the pain associated with it, let me show you how I have and more importantly how you can overcome stuttering to live a fulfilled life. If you feel like you have not fulfilled your potential at work, or in your social life then this is about to change with this book.

This will not be a painless quick journey for you but the word which I will emphasise to you again and again is "perseverance". It will be worth all the effort when you can talk fluently and have the confidence that goes along with that.

What I am about to give you is not only a few breathing exercises or techniques but a complete holistic approach to overcoming your stuttering, starting from your inner being moving towards practical advice. As a parent I also wanted this book to contain advice specifically targeted at treating children. So whether you are a stutterer, a parent of a child that stutters or a loved one that is concerned about someone that stutters, this is the book for you.

When I mention that I spent a huge majority of my life struggling with a stutter problem to people who don't know me, they are surprised and shocked to say the least. A lot of them think I'm having them on and it's some sort of joke. Why is that? Because I speak fluently! I know you may find it difficult to believe but it is true and I am going to share with you how I did it throughout this book.

Before I begin on how I used my holistic approach to treating stuttering, I have to point out I overcame stuttering without the need of medication, any devices or any other methods which give you hope but nothing changes or you realise it's only a short term fix. When all you want is something to work long term right? I have never heard of anyone who has managed to become fluent permanently by using those techniques.

Ok, there are two very important things. The first thing is that I struggled with a stuttering problem for over 30 years. Now that's a long time. My life would have been so different if I spoke the way I do now.

Anyway the second thing is that a few years ago I managed to cure my stuttering after working out some very crucial things about why I stuttered. I know how painful it is to go through life stuttering, the problems you face daily as I've been there myself.

I am just aiming to help others feel the way I do by helping you set yourself free in the world of speech.

I do not believe I am unique or special in any way whatsoever. I believe the way I overcame stuttering, anyone else out there suffering from this problem can do the same. You can see a huge increase in your fluency and with time you can overcome it the way I did. I want to make one thing very clear before I begin to get into the nitty gritty of how I overcame stuttering.

If you are looking for a quick fix then this is not your answer. This is not a miracle cure, I am sorry to disappoint you. They don't exist and until they do you have my method. Don't give up until you've given it a go!!

I want you to know that while I think that many of you reading this book will see some results quite quickly, it will entail some hard work on your part if you want to succeed. I know people want immediate gratification but I have no interest in joining the list of people who offer miracle cures that do not work. I have spent hundreds of pounds on these types of methods on my mission to overcome stuttering and I know how frustrating and heart breaking it all is which is why I want to save you this pain.

I know many of you will have your doubts. You may think that the same method which worked for me can't work for you. You may even doubt that I really overcame it and if you heard me speak fluently you may question if I ever had a stuttering problem to start with. I know precisely why you may be having these doubts.

You have been told time after time that you cannot overcome stuttering that you've started to believe it. You have been told there is no cure and you have to learn to deal with it and manage the best you can.

Well I am here to destroy that belief of yours! The only reason you have been told the same thing over and over again is because no one has been able to come up with something that would work long term for stuttering. Which is why the speech therapists, who are the so called 'experts' in stuttering have proclaimed stuttering as an incurable disability. They are the experts, which is why we believe what they tell us. That's where it all goes wrong.

We believe them to the point where we don't have room for doubt in our minds. If we did then maybe more of us would try to help ourselves but instead of that we just feel helpless about the whole situation.

Well I am living proof that they are wrong!! They can argue with me all they want about it not being possible to overcome stuttering but they can't argue with me that I have not overcome it because I have. The people who know me know I'm living proof of this and I want to share with you how I overcame stuttering.

I honestly want to help you reach a life where your day is stutter free. Before I share all that with you, I'd like to tell you a little about myself and how I struggled with stuttering for the best part of my life.

About Me

I had a stutter from as far back as I can remember. Feelings of isolation, frustration and at times anger compounded the usual anxieties of early childhood and adolescence. People look at me today, successful, confident, and articulate; with everything I want or need. Who would believe I was such a withdrawn child and spent much of my formative years being bullied at school, barely being able to say my name fluently.

I knew I had a problem that prevented me from fitting in, but why I had it or how I could make it go away was a total mystery, that neither I, nor anyone around me could explain.

Visiting the speech therapist with my 5 year old son - who also has a stutter – made me think back to when I was his age and was first taken to the speech therapist.

29 years later, times have changed considerably and while there's certainly a lot more knowledge, awareness and understanding out there, does that mean anything to a five year old? A child who cannot comprehend why he struggles to communicate as fluently as other children in his class, or the children he plays with? It's perhaps therefore unsurprising that when the speech therapist asked my son why he thinks he stutters, he replied plainly "it's because I don't know how to talk properly". As a parent, hearing my child voice his insecurity in such a resigned and factual manner was pretty heartbreaking to say the least. At five years old, my son already felt different and slightly isolated because of a speech impediment. Thinking back to when I was his age, I can relate to those frustrations. Early school reports diagnosed me as having dyslexia; while others routinely pointed

to the barriers I faced because of my 'speech impediment'.

To make matters worse, I was constantly bullied throughout school and as a result became very shy and withdrawn. Some days were worse than others. There were times when I couldn't even say my own name; four simple letters - A.B.I.D - would throw me into a nervous fix, struggling, trying to force out the words. Simple things like that were incredibly challenging for me, and my only response was to hide away.

None of it made any sense and no one seemed to have an explanation or answers.

I was sent to a speech therapist whilst I was at primary school. I would go every 2 weeks with my father and sit in the cold room with this strange woman who would talk to me as if I had just landed from Mars. I would always wonder why she is speaking to me in super slow motion.

Anyway she advised me to speak more slowly – overlooking the glaringly obvious that I already communicated at a painfully slow pace; she introduced me to the novel idea of speaking in rhythm that I should sound out my words like the ticking of a clock.

As you can imagine, my new style of speech did not go amiss amongst my school fellows.

Tick tock, tick tock...yes I sounded like a malfunctioning cyborg, much to the amusement of the other kids. I later discovered that speaking in rhythm was actually a really good tool that could have helped me reduce my stutter but she did not know how to communicate this to me.

Just like most parents of stutterers my family were very concerned about my dysfluency. I was the first person in my entire family including my army of extended family to have a stutter.

My mother had this notion that if she fed me almonds I would stop stuttering, some Asian old wives tale. I was fed almonds for breakfast, lunch and dinner! As you can imagine I cannot stand the sight of them now.

The transition from primary to secondary school is a pretty daunting prospect from most 11 year olds, but the fact that my dad had opted to send me to a Roman Catholic school - where I was one of three Muslim children in the entire school- made it a somewhat more terrifying transition. Here I faced the ultimate double handicap, not only did I stutter but I was a Muslim – both worked against me at my school and the bullying continued.

I must have been 12 years old, when my dad suggested one day that he could come into my school and speak to my teachers about my situation. The mere thought of my dad intervening filled me with dread,

'What would the other children think of me'? But I'd always trusted my dad and had faith in his wisdom.

Before I could offer any protest, he added, "It might help you for a few days but then it'll still be bad, so you're going to have to deal with it at some point". My dad couldn't offer me a treatment or cure, but his constant love, guidance and presence empowered me in a way that I felt blessed to have someone so special in my life. My dad was my only source of comfort and strength through the most difficult and joyous times of my life and he remains so, to this day.

First year of college was quite difficult, but I'd started to explore ways of controlling my stutter. I tried to breathe more slowly when speaking, because I'd run out of breath when talking.

Moving onto University was another huge challenge; I still hadn't been able to get a grip on my stuttering but I was determined not to let it hold me back. My dad had instilled enough confidence in me for me to know that I would overcome this one day and in spite of the stutter make a success of my life. It was great meeting so many different people and I very much enjoyed the social life at university.

Around this time I started observing how other people spoke, especially people on TV, John Snow on the Channel 4 News, even Dr Phil from Oprah; it sounds funny now, but I'd carefully watch how they spoke and accentuated their words and then try out those techniques myself.

By the second year of university I felt more confident and was beginning to develop ways and techniques of controlling my stuttering. I had some great friends, who may not have fully understood the challenges I faced, but never treated me differently because of my stuttering.

More importantly, they would never finish off my sentences, this may sound like a mute point, but it's a common tendency for people to finish off sentences for people who speak slowly or with any kind of speech impediment and they think they are doing you a favour. When in actual fact it can be very demoralizing.

Increasing confidence coupled with age and experience certainly helped, but that's not to say I found a miracle cure, I just got better at finding coping strategies and techniques. But it was still a struggle and I had to work twice as hard to get by. I remember having to deliver a presentation in my second year of university, to my tutors and approximately 30 other students.

I couldn't sleep for days beforehand and my anxiety levels were soaring to the point where I was physically sick. On the day itself, my hands were shaking and at some point I couldn't feel my feet or legs. Admittedly it was now a familiar feeling; I went through the same angst during my GCSE English oral exam, which incidentally I failed miserably.

At the age of 15 I remember vividly having to deliver a presentation at a Mosque and I froze, I knew what I had to say, but my brain and mouth failed to comply, leaving me vulnerable to the taunts of my class fellow and more frightfully the unrelenting Mosque teacher, who refused to show any hint of compassion towards the mumbling child frozen in the centre of the room. I cried on my way home from Mosque that day.

Securing a job with the NHS as a newly qualified podiatrist was a dream come true for me, seeing the joy I could bring to patients was an absolute joy for me. Interestingly enough, I would rarely stutter when speaking with patients. Yet with colleagues, I would still stutter with most of my words. But I never allowed this to dull my self-belief and ambition.

I vividly remember an incident when I had to visit a patient at home for a home visit; I turned up and knocked on the door.

The door opened and I had to ask for this patient, I suffered a severe block and could not get the name of the patient out. The woman's daughter came to the door and started pointing at me and laughing, by this stage the woman also had a huge smirk on her face.

I could feel more anxiety building up inside me and wishing the earth would open up and swallow me up. When I eventually got her name out she informed me that it was her sister and she wasn't home.

As I returned back to the car and sat on my own for a few minutes, I felt as though I had been spat at or sworn at but it was just someone laughing at my stutter. The rest of that day went by with the image of that lady and her daughter pointing and laughing at me.

I eventually left the NHS and my lucrative private practice that I had developed over the years to fulfil a dream or vision I had in my head, which was to set up an Internet foot care products website. When I told everyone what I was going to do I got the same reaction as when I told them about this book, they laughed and doubted I could do it.

This was the only motivation I needed and I worked very hard to learn a completely new set of skills such as web design, programming and how to run a business. The business is now worth 5 million pounds and I have achieved many of the things I wanted to in relation to the business. I have had business meetings over the years when I was very conscious about my stuttering; in fact it reminded me of being at school again.

However now I have developed a holistic approach to stuttering and I can speak completely fluently. I'm not going to say it was easy as it was far from easy, but just like developing my own online business, nothing of great value comes easily in life.

I really want to share with you the system I have developed over the years and how you can start to make your first steps towards fluency.

I'm absolutely sure that if you follow this book you can overcome your stuttering and lead a productive life filled with joy and happiness. What you will not get from this book is a medical based journal with the use of jargon and more importantly negativity. I'm going to write this from the heart and in a way that I hope everyone can read, understand and implement what I have discovered.

So Why Me?

Stuttering has been around for centuries with the differing views concerning the causes and treatment of stuttering. In ancient Greece, theories referred to dryness of the tongue. In the 19th century, abnormalities of the speech apparatus were thought to cause stuttering. Thus, treatment was based on extensive "plastic" surgery, often leading to mutilations and additional disabilities. Other treatment options were tongue weights or mouth prostheses. At present there are over 55 million people around the world that stutter, so if you are a stutterer you are not alone.

The Gender Link

Gender is one of the strongest predisposing factors for stuttering in that the disorder affects many more males than females. So why are us boys being discriminated against so heavily by nature? It has been widely debated if nurture i.e. the environment you have been bought up in or nature are responsible for stuttering. Most conditions are probably a mixture of both, as languages and culture are dependent upon your environment and conditions can be heredity.

The stuttering disorder gap between the genders increases for 3 year olds, which is at a ratio of 2:1 to 4:1 for adults. That's four men for every 1 woman that stutters!

This sex ratio discrimination is also present for a variety of other conditions such as autism and learning difficulties.

Research has shown that women and men's brains are different! All the women in my life are going to have a broad smile on their faces right now as I constantly hear "man bashing" in my household. Anyway back to the point, women's brains are more resilient as they recover from strokes quicker.

Also evidence from brain imaging has shown that women tend to have a thicker corpus callosum (part of the brain that affects speech) than men. Girls that stutter tend to have a higher recovery rate and better compensation techniques.

It is evident that nurture is more to blame than nature. The environment in which you are brought up in can affect your recovery but not necessarily cause your stuttering.

Research has suggested that children that are bought up in bilingual families are at greater risk of developing this condition as the child's brain has to process the complexities of two languages. It has not been proven that these children in multi-linguistic and multicultural families would not have developed a stutter if they were in a monolingual household but it can prove to be a trigger.

The Neurological Link

Studies have been carried out using positron emission tomography (PET) to scan the brain of stutterers and fluent people to make observations. It was discovered that stutterers tend to use the right side of their brain more than fluent people. The left side of the brain is responsible for speech, but it is being interrupted by the right side when speaking.

Some professionals think that stress can actually cause stuttering. When visiting a sp60eech therapist with my son I was repeatedly asked if he had experienced any traumatic event in the family when he first started talking. This got me thinking that there must be a link between a traumatic experience and stuttering. However after doing extensive research it is not possible to say this categorically.

Some children go through traumatic experiences and do not develop a stutter while others do. Stutterers do have higher levels of social anxiety but stress is a trigger for stuttering but not necessarily a cause of stuttering.

Neural activation patterns were observed of stutterers and fluent people and it was confirmed that stutterers do bias the right side of their brain more compared to fluent people. An interesting fact is that 50-80% of children that stutter overcome the condition with treatment.

However PET scans have revealed that children like me that continued stuttering into adulthood have decreased auditory cortex and hyperactivity of the speech centre. The problem with using neural studies to study the cause of stuttering is that the neural system is responsible for human behaviour. Everyone has unique behavioural traits and life experiences that can affect the neural system. Why does stuttering cause a different part of the brain to be active? There is a theory called the valsalva mechanism. This is a natural body function that involves the lungs creating pressure by forcefully closing the upper airway at the same time the chest and abdominal muscles contract.

Ordinarily the Valsalva manoeuvre (with its accompanying effort of the closure of the voice box) is done instinctively, without conscious thought.

This occurs in normal, healthy people during lifting, pushing, pulling, defecation, natural childbirth, and other strenuous tasks. The reason why this is connected to stuttering is that when we stutterers talk, we put a lot of effort into the words that we are trying to say. Fluent speaking people require a minimum of effort to talk; when stutterers talk they put a lot of effort in the valsalva mechanism which causes tightness of the larynx (voice box). People who stutter may have learned to activate the Valsalva mechanism in an effort to produce words, as if they were things to be forced out of the body. Such activation is most likely to occur when the stutterer anticipates difficulty or feels the need to use extra effort to speak properly.

While this might instinctively feel like the right thing to do, it actually makes fluent speech impossible.

This mechanism is connected neurologically and therefore can be connected to a neurological component of speech. Let's link all of this in relatively plain English, let's say a stutterer wants to say "ninety nine". The stutterer may know from previous experiences that the letter "n" will be hard to say so the brain recognises this and the valsalva mechanism is activated and therefore shuts air in the lungs and tightens the voice box.

The more I examined the neurological causes of stuttering the more I knew that the key to curing stuttering was to re-train your brain.

I will explain how to do that in the next chapter but the fact that scientists agree that the mind and not the body is the problem was fascinating. It started me on a journey to understand why the brain behaves like this and if I could cure my own stuttering.

I've spent so much time reading articles, books, stuttering blogs, where all I would come across was negativity, "let's do more research into stuttering" and it can be "controlled" with help. I would never hear anyone say it can be cured as people would not even consider it as a possibility. The people that know me will testify that I never give up no matter how hard the task before me is so now armed with the research I started to develop my own holistic approach to curing my stutter.

It's all in your Mind

Blame

Throughout my life I was determined to learn the best skills I could to try to minimise my stuttering problem as much as possible. I used to constantly look at other people talking and try to notice why they could talk fluently and I couldn't. I couldn't find any books on stuttering at those times. I didn't realise there was such a lack of information out there. From what I did find though, I quickly started to realise that the experts didn't know what caused stuttering and I wasn't going to find any answers from learning how it begins.

This is something that you really need to take in. You should not waste valuable time accessing your childhood to try and find out whom or what is to blame. I tried to do that and I achieved nothing from it. My parents would tell me that I developed my stutter after going away on holiday and falling ill; as I got older I realised that stuttering is not a disease that you can catch like malaria. But for years I blamed this holiday. Take my advice; leave the past in the past. Sometimes people blame stuttering because of a traumatic event which has taken place. Forget about who should be blamed. Forget about blaming your family, or moaning about your parents not reading to you.

Stop trying to work out if it's hereditary or not, it's not going to change anything. In your mind stop focusing on trying to work out if you have a physical defect in your speaking mechanism or what you did wrong to add to your speech problem. None of this helps. I'm astounded at how often people blame everything that goes wrong in their lives on others, focusing on the cause of stuttering just causes negative energy. You need to fill your mind with positive thoughts and avoid blaming yourself.

Studies

As I've mentioned in the previous chapters, I was always fascinated by the studies which showed people who stutter have different brain scans than a person who does not stutter.

To begin with I was confused to say the least and I started wondering whether the experts were right after all. How can someone overcome stuttering when the studies show that a part of the brain or speaking mechanism is different or even 'abnormal' in a person who stutters? How can you argue with evidence like that? Doesn't that prove that there is a physical defect in a person who stutters? Doesn't that make it impossible to overcome?

After doing more research things started to look clearer to me. They started to make sense. It was clear why someone who stutters would have a different brain scan to someone who doesn't. It was obvious that some physical component of our speech mechanism or a part of our brain would look like it was damaged or different.
There's no way that both brains could be the same, it was impossible for them to be different.

The reason behind this doesn't have to be because of a defect or a flaw, it's simply because internal conditions are always shown externally. The problem is on the inside but on the outside a person will stutter.

We all know that stress leads to all kinds of physical problems right? Such as heart attacks, headaches, ulcers and so on. You can treat any of these symptoms but unless you treat the root cause which in this case is stress, you will carry on suffering with physical problems. Let me give you an example, we all know that congestive heart failure can be caused by smoking, so you need to find the underlying cause and treat it otherwise you'll never be rid of it. This is the same for stuttering, if you do not address the root cause, you'll never be free from stuttering. Physical symptoms can be relieved temporarily but they will always continue to come back until the root cause is treated. You can cover a problem up with a plaster but as soon as you rip it off the problem is still there.

Make your Intention

Ok now I want you to take a minute to make your intention in your mind that stuttering can be overcome. If you find it hard to do this because of all the rubbish the 'experts' have fed you over all those years then at least tell yourself that the 'experts' can be wrong. Once your mind has registered that, keep telling yourself that you can overcome stuttering.

If you make it into a possibility then it has more of a chance of coming true. It is vital that you do this. Making an intention is an essential mental step as it will pave the path for you to cure your stuttering problem.

I've always had self-belief that I could fix my own stuttering problem. There's always going to be people who will say you can't overcome it. That's when you go into a negative mindset. You need to overcome that barrier and believe that you can overcome stuttering to the point where it happens.

Another thing which let me know that I could overcome stuttering was when I noticed my external stuttering pattern wasn't the same all the time. What I mean is that in different situations I'd stutter on different words. I may stutter on the word 'won't' in one situation but in a different situation the word 'won't' would come out perfectly. I was also intrigued over why I stuttered at school and not in front of my sisters. This got me thinking; if I really had a physical problem then I wouldn't be able to say the word 'won't' any of the time. Take a moment and think about it. Why is it that sometimes you can say a word perfectly and another time you'll stutter on the same word? This was something I just had to find out.

Thoughts

One day I came across a series of books which changed my whole outlook on stuttering. I was never a great reader but when I came across one book, I wanted to read more books and take in as much information as I could. That sent me searching in a new direction altogether to discover what I needed to overcome stuttering.

I guess you're all wondering what it was? Well basically it's your thoughts! Everyone has individual personalities, their own self image, there's even a success mechanism, and all of these come from your head, from your thoughts!

I would never have thought that my thoughts could be having such a major and important part in my stuttering problem until I read those books. Since then I have read countless books on the topic. I also have studied how the brain functions, that's the only way I could understand how my brain works and what part is linked with my thoughts. I had to know how my thought process was linked to my stuttering. I was astonished about what I learnt.

Not only did I discover that my thoughts played a major part in my problem but also that my thought process was going to play an enormous part in me overcoming stuttering.

What you spend your time thinking about is what you'll sooner or later end up creating in your life, or attracting to yourself. It is known as the Law of Attraction. Whether or not you realise it you are always thinking, if you're speaking to others, listening, watching the television or reading a paper you are thinking. When you are driving you are thinking about other things and even when you wake up first thing in the morning to brush your teeth your mind is on hyper drive thinking about what your next step will be. Your thoughts attract what you are thinking about to yourself. They have an effect on your everyday life. You'll be amazed at how powerful your own thoughts are and how they affect you.

Why do you think 1% of the population earn 96% of the worlds wealth. People draw whatever they want into their lives whether it is wealth, love, happiness or fluency through the law of attraction. The wealthy people's prominent thoughts are about an abundance of wealth and they do not allow negative thoughts to enter into their minds, by doing this whether knowingly or unknowingly they can attract further wealth but using the law of attraction. The simplest way of looking at the law is to think of yourself as the most powerful magnet in the universe and you will attract everything you want or don't want through your thoughts.

This concept has not just been discovered, it's been around for centuries. Some of the most influential people throughout history have spoken about the law such as Shakespeare, Beethoven, Leonardo Di Vinci, Socrates, Plato, Isaac Newton to mention a few. The law of attraction has been described by Charles Haanel in 1912 "...the greatest and most infallible law".

Your thoughts act like a magnet and attract other thoughts on the same frequency. If you are complaining about something the law of attraction will bring you more situations you have to complain about. You can see the law of attraction everywhere; you draw circumstances, jobs, people, relationships, debt and joy towards you through your thoughts. It is indiscriminate so whatever you think about you attract.

Have you ever got angry or thought about something that upset you? Did you notice that the more you thought about it the more upset you got? Or have you heard a song on the radio that you couldn't get out of your head. This is because that at that time you gave that song or sad thought your full attention, you were attracting similar thoughts. Now you may not understand how this law of attraction works but that doesn't mean it doesn't exist. When you switch the light switch on and your room becomes bright you don't know how exactly the electricity was generated and transferred to your home but you know you have light! That is the same with the law of attraction. Out thoughts produce a frequency that attracts similar frequencies.

I'm sure that the majority of us do not understand the impact our thoughts have on us on a daily basis. It's all to do with positive energy. Each thought is a form of creation especially if it is accompanied by feelings, it attracts other thoughts. Positive thoughts attract positive thoughts and negative thoughts attract negative thoughts. You'll have to be aware of your thoughts to be able to change them from disempowering thoughts to empowering thoughts. This is vital to overcome stuttering.

To help you become more attentive of your thoughts, ask yourself during the day how do I feel? Do I expect to be fluent or to stutter when I speak today? Do I expect the worst possible outcome? Do I have to think ahead to establish which words are going to be a problem for me? How do I think others see me?

Do you tend to think that you will never be able to overcome stuttering, you will never be able to speak fluently or get anywhere in life because you have a speech impediment? Do you tell yourself that you are powerless and that you can't do anything about your stuttering? Have you ever made those statements to yourself about yourself?

You have to start being aware of these types of thoughts and then begin to change them. It is not impossible to break down your existing thought pattern and change it to a more empowering way of thinking, a more improved way. To begin with I would like you to start noticing when you have a negative thought about stuttering. To do this you just have to start observing your own thoughts. This will feel weird to begin with and even maybe a little tricky and hard too but don't give up. It'll get easier with a little practice and before you know it you will be an expert in spotting negative thoughts.

Visualization

Visualization is a powerful exercise, as you create pictures in your mind about your fluency; you are generating positive emotions and attracting a positive fluent frequency. When you visualize your fluency it will materialise. I've always had a picture in my head of whatever I've wanted in life and I would focus on that constantly, not letting negative thoughts creep into my mind. This attracted positive energy and opportunities came to me when I wasn't expecting them.

When you focus on your fluency you will attract positive vibrations and you will accomplish your goals. The feelings you generate create the attraction not just the thought of you being fluent, you have to actually believe it, and you have to visualize talking fluently and feel how good it feels in your heart. You could do this daily and use vivid visualizations rather than static.
Let me give you an example, close your eyes, imagine opening the door which has a cold handle. As you walk into the room you see everyone you love and care about sitting down waiting for you to give a talk.

As you walk to the front you say hello to your friends and smile and give one of your friends a little wink of the eye to tell her you're ok.

You then walk up to the front and crack a small joke to make people laugh. You then proceed to give a speech about a topic that interests you, completely fluently without stuttering or blocking even once. That's vivid visualization and the benefits of it are immense.

I also want you to think of a positive thought that fills you with joy, in my case it's watching my son play football. Write that positive thought down and other things related to stuttering, for instance the word 'fluency' or I would write "I can talk fluently" on small pieces of paper and stick them next to your bed, office, in your car and in your sitting room so that you are constantly reminded about them.

I would stick up a piece of paper on the ceiling of the bedroom so as soon as I woke up and looked up I would be reminded of being fluent which would fill me with joy! I want you to also go through a 15 minute meditation process everyday. People think you have to be up some mountain, where birds are singing to do meditation.

That is not the case, you can do it anywhere even in a traffic jam. Think about being fluent, visualise it so that you can turn that image into reality. One more thing I want you to do is talk as much as you can to your family and friends, give talks about what you're interested in, whether it's cooking, cars, even brick-laying if that's what you're into.

It is important to be grateful for what you have; this will stop you from constantly focusing on your stutter and bring about positive emotions which will act like a magnet to attract other positive emotions. Focus on what you do have and be thankful for it, I would typically wake up and start the day off with my "gratitude routine". You may think this is really whishy washy and has got nothing to do with stuttering but setting the mood in your mind is so important. It's like making dinner for a loved one; you may light a candle and play some slow background music to set the mood for the dinner. Being consciously grateful and saying thank you for everything you have sets the mood for your mind to think positively. You can carry this through the day so if you have arrived at your destination you can be grateful for getting there in one piece.

What if I don't believe the law of attraction, will it still affect me?

Of course it will. You are offering vibrations and sending out positive or negative energy by default, you have been doing it ever since you came to understand your environment. Not understanding the law is like driving a car without knowing the rules of the road. You're going to end up somewhere you don't want to be or even worse you're going to have a crash. Knowing about the law gives you the knowledge to be able to gain control over your life.

Can I change the momentum of my thoughts from the past?

You have been thinking about stuttering ever sense you started talking and you realised that you were different from other people. These thoughts have created a momentum by the law of attraction. Whatever you think about, you draw more similar things towards you until the negative bundle of energy gets bigger and bigger. The feelings that you have about stuttering have caused a gradual momentum and you need to change the direction of your thoughts towards fluency. Start to think about thoughts, about fluency, and start off by thinking about being fluent in certain circumstances such as ordering food in a restaurant.

Also start to look at the positive aspects of your life such as having a good job, caring family, house that you can call home. This will change the momentum of your thoughts that have been built up over the years towards a positive direction.

Receiving

An important part of the law of attraction is the ability to receive. Feel how good it feels to be fluent. Believe you are already fluent; get the feeling of the fluent frequency. Let's say you won the lottery today and you knew you were going to get a large cheque in a weeks time, you would have the reassurance that the money was coming and you would have that feeling in the pit of your stomach. That's the feeling I want you to develop about your fluency. You not only have to think about being fluent but have the emotional intensity that accompanies that thought, that's when your thoughts are giving you power to help you accomplish anything.

It also makes life easier once you accept that you are fluent, imagine yourself white water rafting against the current, and now imagine rowing with the current. That is the feeling of receiving, it's so much easier.

You may ask how long it is going to take for me to recover from my stutter using these methods. As quantum physicists will tell you, everything is happening at once and a parallel fluent version of you already exists!

Any delay in you getting to the fluent
state is your inability of being, knowing
and feeling fluency. Now you may be
like me, constantly asking questions
looking for scientific proof of everything
before you can believe in a theory.

There is so much in this world and in the
universe that we don't know about. Let
me give you a few examples,
astronomers know that the universe is
expanding rapidly but cannot
understand why it is as it should
according to our laws of science be
slowing down. Time only goes in one
direction so everyone gets old,
according to physicists it should be
symmetrical. For me, what the most
astounding unknowns about the
universe is dark matter and dark energy.

The vast majority of the universe is made
up of this dark energy and dark matter;
we don't know its origin or its
composition. It's not even dark! It's

transparent, and adds to the weight of the universe.

Astronomers know about the big bang theory but they are still at a loss to know what happened just before the big bang. The big bang created hydrogen, helium and lithium which are what we are made up of and can interact with light. But why is our planet the only one blessed with this in our universe? I know this may sound like a science lesson but it's important to understand that we cannot explain everything in this universe and so should have an open mind.

From a medical point of view trials using a placebo and actual medication often produce the same results. Patients actually get cured from a disease because they think and more importantly believe that they will be cured even though there is nothing in the medication they are taking. When I was a student I used to always wonder why on earth this would happen. At that time I couldn't comprehend the power of the mind and the healing qualities associated with it.

There are numerous examples of cancer patients getting miracle cures which cannot be explained from a medical perspective. This is what the power of the mind can accomplish.

Healing through the mind can cure your stuttering! I'm absolutely sure of this but it is important you "think perfect fluency".

Writing

If you ask any stutterer to describe what emotions they are experiencing, they may say fear, anxiety, anger but you will never hear someone describing stuttering as fun. Actually facing up to your emotions about stuttering is not such as bad thing. The distinction between facing up to your emotions and recognising them and making them the primary focus in your life is huge. Remember your primary focus should be "effective communication" Being able to face up to all the negative emotions is the first step in eliminating stuttering. Being honest with yourself about your fears and anxieties sows the ground for effective fluency.

A good way of doing this is to write all your feelings about stuttering down on paper. You can write them by recalling painful experiences or you could write a fictional story and almost observe the life of a stutterer from above. I personally wrote all my feelings about my stuttering down on paper and buried them in the garden. This was not my way of hiding my emotions but of me facing up to them and moving on from them. I was no longer going to feel "abnormal" and a "defect" as these feelings were buried away in the garden and were no longer a part of my life.

The process of writing can also be used by teenagers that are suffering from bullying at school due to their stuttering.

It will help parents and teachers to understand what is going on as the teenager may not have the confidence to physically tell someone. As a parent one of the biggest fears is that a child gets bullied to such as extent that they consider self harm. Providing a way in which they can vent their anger and release their emotions is essential to prevent a teenager feeling alone and desperate. When I was bullied at school due to my stuttering I felt very lonely and I would often be in tears on the way back from school.

However, I was lucky to have such an understanding father who would constantly reassure me.

Writing and reading stories in which characters can overcome adversities can also be inspirational.

Stuttering is often made worse by the anxiety about situations and the trepidation of problem words or sounds. For instance I know that I may get stuck when saying my first name, Abid as I get stuck on "a's". I found reading and writing stories that would involve a character facing up to and defeating his fears inspirational.

Stuttering Pattern

To overcome stuttering I had to observe my own stuttering patterns thoroughly. I was examining the smallest of thoughts. I was fascinated by the fact that I could speak fluently in some situations but I was an utter mess in others. Why was it that I was absolutely fluent when I was speaking to my family?

I started to concentrate on every part of my stuttering. This took up a lot of energy as it's very hard to focus. You have to concentrate very hard and you should be prepared for that too. It can be quite draining to begin with. Like I have said before, this is not a miracle cure; it requires complete dedication on your part. Just keep telling yourself it'll be worth it in the long run. It all depends on how much you really want to stop stuttering. If you want it bad enough then no obstacle or hard work can get in your way. You just need the right attitude, if you believe you can and will overcome stuttering then you will.

It worked for me and there's no reason whatsoever why it shouldn't work for you. I won't lie to you, I had to work very hard to get to where I am today and if you put in the same hard work and dedication then you will see the results you want.

It definitely isn't easy to begin with and you will feel like giving up but hang in there, remind yourself why you are doing this. Exposing and trying to reveal subconscious thoughts, behaviours and beliefs is not something we usually do so to begin with our brains will struggle and try to refuse to go on with this exercise. Stick with it and it'll come around.

Stuttering just seems to happen, it can happen at any time. We rarely take the time to analyze our stuttering patterns. This is exactly what I'm asking you to do now. Try to notice when, where, how and why you are stuttering. Write it down. Make a note of everything you become aware of when you are stuttering. Is there a pattern? Note down how you are feeling before, during and after you speak. Were you excited? Fearful? Anxious? Nervous? Sick? Fretful? Restless? Write down absolutely everything. Write down what you were thinking before, during and after you spoke? What was going on inside your head when you spoke? Write that down too. All this is crucial because it will help you discover a lot about yourself. You will be amazed to say the least at what you find out.

It is vital to help you reveal your subconscious behaviour, beliefs and values. When I first began to do this, I was astonished by what I discovered. I had no idea what was behind my stuttering most of the time and I could have gone through the rest of my life not knowing had I not started to dig in and spend time discovering information about myself.

I spent months totally immersed in working out what my stuttering pattern was, all that hard work paid off as now I had a strong base to help me with the rest of the things I had to do to overcome stuttering. Just by discovering my stuttering patterns greatly reduced the amount of stuttering as I progressed. The reason why is simple, it's because for the first time in my life I knew what was making me stutter. I actually consciously knew why I was stuttering in particular situations and this gave me the opportunity to reassess the root cause.

I will give you an example to explain what I mean. After I started to observe my own stuttering patterns, one of the first things that I noticed was that I found it very hard to speak fluently with authority figures.

An authority figure can be anyone, a friend, teacher or a mentor. Anyone you feel is better than you in a better way. Working that out and being aware of that fact was just the beginning. After that I had to search even more, dig deeper to work out what it was about authority figures which left me the way it did, in such a predicament! This took a lot of effort and attention. Knowing that authority figures had an effect on me when I spoke was just the start; it was just like scratching the surface. I had to go below that to have a chance of removing this part of stuttering in my speech.

The things I discovered which concerned authority figures and my unconscious thoughts about them at the start were that I thought they were cleverer and smarter than I was. Their opinion about me was correct.

They would judge me by the way I spoke; they are in a higher position so they have power over me. I even thought what they think of me makes me who I am and if I'm worth anything or not.

When I started thinking about authority figures, I had no idea that all these thoughts and feelings were linked to the causes of stuttering when speaking to authority figures. On a conscious level, I had no idea all that was going on in my head. Why is that? When you start thinking about something normally and it becomes natural then sooner or later it will move into your subconscious and run automatically. You wouldn't even need to think about it, it would just happen.

Once I had figured out what my thoughts and beliefs were about authority figures, I completely understood why speaking with them was so hard. Even more importantly, I was able to reassess my thoughts and beliefs to see if they were in fact true or not. I will be telling you about this a little further on. For now though, I want you to get a note book and begin to observe your own stuttering patterns over the next couple of weeks.

Every time you stutter I would like you to write down who you were speaking to when you stuttered? What were you feeling at the time? (fearful, nervous, unsure, insecure, anxious, sick?) What was the subject you were discussing or topic you were talking about? Remember, this is an important part of the process in becoming fluent. Please do not blow it off, ignore it or miss it out. What you put into this step is exactly what you will get out of it.

When you have spent a few weeks observing your stuttering patterns then go back and take a look at your note book and try to notice the patterns. You will have patterns; I have no doubt about that. You may have already noticed a number of those patterns by now. I want you to really go through your note book with precision and find every incident where the same event or feeling took place a number of times, at least 3 times or more. These are your patterns, also known as 'trigger' points. Each person has different trigger points.

You can't treat all stutterers the same, they are individuals. People tend to think that the same thing will set a stutterer off, if only it was that simple. If that was the case, then stutterers could avoid those things and never worry about stuttering again. I will tell you what to do with trigger points a little further on.

Your Beliefs

First I think I need to talk to you a little about beliefs. You might be thinking why beliefs would have a role in the recovery process. Well I can tell you that beliefs have a huge part in the recovery process.

One of the most powerful mechanisms are beliefs, this mechanism works throughout the entire day. Your brain is unable to take in all the data we give it every single second, minute and hour of everyday in your life.

For that reason, it has to filter the data it receives and only let a certain amount come into your conscience and finally into your subconscious. Beliefs are one of the main ways your brain knows what to let in and what to get rid of.

This mechanism used for filtering in your brain looks at your present beliefs and then whatever data it receives from the outside world has to match your beliefs before it will let the data become a part of your conscience, meaning a part of your reality.

I'll give you an example. At a subconscious level you may have developed a belief that all Muslims are terrorists and horrible people after 9/11 and 7/7 or you may believe that all men with beards are terrorists but a friend of yours or a neighbour may know a Muslim and they might believe that they are good people. This is when you start to filter dealings with Muslims according to your beliefs. You will take into account all the things you hear on the news or in the papers, which will reconfirm your belief that all Muslims are terrorists, even though you know that the news only talks about a minority not the majority of Muslims.

But what if most of the people you knew thought Muslims were good people? The odds are you would probably disagree with them and carry on believing that all Muslims are terrorists. Why do you think your beliefs would be so different from everyone else you knew? You've probably been able to guess by now. It's because you are filtering information based on your belief that all Muslims are terrorists and horrible people.

You notice everything bad about them whereas other people are filtering the data according to their own beliefs which could be opposite to what you believe. They may be filtering every kind and caring act whereas you are filtering every unkind act.

It is fascinating because you and your friends or neighbours are living in the same town or city amongst the same people but what you think about Muslims is absolutely different compared to each other. This is when an interesting question arises. Who is right and who is wrong? Can there be a right and wrong in this situation?

Think about it. Think about your family and your siblings. You and your brothers and sisters were bought up in the same environment but are you not all unique?

I was bought up with my 5 sisters in the same house but we all turned out differently. They've all got different beliefs when it comes to culture and religion. Some of them are religious and some are not. Bad things have happened in our childhood but everyone found their own way of dealing with them. As for me, the events in my life have made me into the person I am today and I'm happy about that. The way we have interpreted and used the events which have happened in our lives make us what we are, that's how our beliefs are formed. I believe whatever happens, happens for a reason. At the end of the day it all comes down to beliefs. Beliefs are very powerful thoughts!!!

Beliefs are one of the most powerful and important tools you have. You may have come across stories about how people are healed or become sick based on their beliefs. Beliefs affect you physically, emotionally and psychologically.

What makes beliefs so powerful? Your brain is not capable of telling reality and non-reality apart. It is an incredible part of all of us that has the vital job of making sure our reality stays together.

How can it know what will keep it together? Your beliefs, that's how. Your beliefs act like commands which your brain has to carry out. Your brain is designed to keep the reality of the world in tact and one of the best ways to do this is to filter the data it receives from the environment around you based on your beliefs.

This is in fact very good because as you may have already noticed, changing your beliefs can change the way your brain filters which can therefore change your present situation. The trouble is that only a small number of us ever assess our current beliefs to make sure that they are still suitable and are helping us the way we need them to. Most of us usually develop a belief and with time it wonders into our subconscious mind and there it will stay and our conscious will never be aware of it again.

The brain constructs inner beliefs about the world. We're only human, sometimes we get it wrong and sometimes we're lucky and we get it right. Luckily the human brain is capable of changing its system of beliefs very quickly. Therefore beliefs are intelligent which invisibly guide our complicated actions of our lives. Most of our beliefs are developed in childhood and depending on your environment, a lot of us still have those beliefs today. If that is the case then that can be pretty harmful as most of our beliefs at that time were used to form us, they were created to protect us. If you didn't have a perfect childhood then you can be certain that you still don't have those beliefs anymore as your environment has changed. Those beliefs have served their purpose. Since you've become an adult, your beliefs also should have adjusted so that they meet your current needs.

Some of your childhood beliefs have obviously changed on their own as you have got older. Most adults do not believe in Superman or Superwoman (for those of you who think I'm being sexiest!) anymore but when you were a child I bet you still jumped off your bed to prove that they exist. The extra knowledge and insight you gain as you get older will of course change and alter some of your beliefs. Nevertheless, once you become conscious of your current beliefs you will be surprised at how many childhood beliefs are still in action.

You have to remember that just because you have a belief does not make it right. We all know that people believed the world was flat for centuries even though we all know that it's not true. Theories of the world being round would enrage 'flat world' believers. Those who believed the world was round were punished. This is how powerful beliefs are. It makes you who you are, what you will do, where you will go, how you will feel, who and what you will tolerate and how you will interact with other people.

Sometimes beliefs are so powerful that they become a big part of your reality which is why many people will die for what they believe in, in spite of them being right or wrong.

Everyone has different beliefs, even if it's not right people still believe it because it's their belief. Lucky for us we can change our beliefs. I am certain that everyone reading this book has had some sort of strong belief at one time or another which changed as you grew older. Maybe you had some strong religious beliefs which changed over time. Beliefs can be changed; they do change all the time. That's all I'm trying to point out.

How can you change a belief? The way beliefs are most often changed is by your environment and by your experiences in life.

This does not mean you have to wait for a life changing event to take place before you can change your beliefs. Just like you are able to assess your beliefs, the same way you can change them too. When you spend time searching for your current beliefs and then bring them back to your conscious level, you have an amazing opportunity to take a look at them again and decide whether you still believe in them or not. Ask yourself are they serving your needs. If they are not then change them into more empowering beliefs, beliefs which will help you achieve what you want in life. In this case it is fluency.

There's no doubt or question in my mind about why I stuttered in the company of authority figures. How could I not stutter? We all deal with stress in different ways.

It comes out in different forms, some of us get headaches, some get high blood pressure, some get back pain and some stutter. Those of us, who carry stress in our speech, how could we not stutter? Especially when we carry around belief about authority figures which is of no use to us. At least I am aware of my beliefs now. I can re-evaluate them and see if they are still what I need or not.

The procedure used to evaluate current beliefs is pretty simple but a very powerful exercise. I shall tell you what I did when it came to my beliefs on authority figures a little further on.

One of the beliefs I had about authority figures was that they had power over me. I had to assess this to work out whether this was still true now that I am an adult. Rationalise it in your head.

For example, if your authority figure is a friend, ask yourself what can this person do to me? What power do they have over me? It all comes down to your own self-worth about yourself. If you have high self worth then you don't need anyone to tell you what you are or what you can do.

I noticed that some authority figures did have power over me but only a little. No way near as much as I once thought. So in fact the truth was nothing compared to what I had believed for the last 30 years of my life. Putting your beliefs into perspective was like setting yourself free. This is why authority figures do not affect me in the same way anymore like they once did.

I shall talk you through another example just to make sure you understand properly. One of the other beliefs that I had was that authority figures made me who I am and they determined what I was worth as a person. As children our authority figures are our parents. It's up to our parents to set our values and define who we are. Our parents' job is to help their children by showing them how valuable they are as human beings. At the end of the day it's up to the environment we are bought up in, we don't all have parents who love us, guide us and help develop us in to decent human beings. On the other hand if you come from a dysfunctional family like most of us do then you usually go into adulthood with a deformed sense of self value.

A normal developmental process would be when a person goes through adolescence and then into adulthood with their beliefs about authority figures decreasing as they grow and gain understanding of their own self-worth.

In my case, my self-worth wasn't much when I was a child but as I grew older it changed. The way you think has a huge impact on your life. Now I have very high self-worth. I know I can do anything if I put my mind to it. It doesn't matter to me if people think I have a big head or I'm full of it. It doesn't matter what other people think of you, what you think is what counts. What matters is that I believe in myself, which is what has got me to where I am today. I have my stutter under control!

Are you starting to see how crucial your beliefs are in getting through your everyday life? If you form beliefs which are empowering then you shall live an empowering life but if you hold on to disempowering beliefs, even childhood beliefs then you will have a lot of things which will get in the way of your everyday life.

You may try and explain to your loved ones that you will cure your stuttering using the techniques in this book and the response may be that of an "unrealistic" expectation. It is important that your thoughts are not influenced by negative comments as it will cause you to have negative thoughts which the law of attraction teaches us will attract greater negativity. When people say "unrealistic" they are forming an image of what "reality" is. They think that their perspective of reality is set in stone and thus affecting your perspective of reality.

Even 5 years ago it would have been "unrealistic" that we could grow back a severed finger with some powder. Well this actually happened this year, a man who lost his fingertip in an accident, grew it back using a powder which was created from a pig bladder lining and left over tissue put in acid.

When I read this for the first time I had to literally pinch myself as I thought it was a wind up but when I realised this study was carried out by Pittsburgh University in the USA it started to make me think about what we humans think about "realistic" expectations.

It would be "unrealistic" to cure your stutter as long as you can only focus on "what is now" you will never be able to see "what is beyond".

You should focus on what you want to see, which is being fluent, I know it's easier said than done but this is a trait that you have to develop to succeed in your fluency.

Now it's your turn. I want you to take your note book out again and look at where you listed your beliefs. Now go through and assess each belief in the same way I did to find out if they are empowering beliefs that you must continue to have. If you notice beliefs that were good for you when you were a child but are useless now that you're an adult then throw them away or bring them up to date so that they can help you now. I was able to look at my list of beliefs that I wrote and straight away I would see the ones which were from my childhood and ones which I had no idea why they were there. A lot of you will be able to do that too.

If you struggle on assessing one or more of your beliefs then do what I did with a number of my beliefs and ask yourself questions. It is an excellent way to filter out unconscious thoughts and feelings.

Your Values

Values are just as important as beliefs. They are easier to understand than beliefs. Values are what hold beliefs together, kind of like glue. A lot of beliefs are in fact created by the values we hold. When one of our values is altered, you can be certain that the belief linked to that value will also change. This is why it is important to look at our current values. It is just as important as understanding our beliefs.

Values are basically defined as what is significant to you. When you have decided what is important to you, you begin to create beliefs or even 'rules' around that value. For example, I value spending time with my son and I believe it is important to do so. As I believe it is important to spend time with my son, I start to create rules around that value. I created a rule like every Saturday morning I would take my son swimming to spend time with him. If I broke one of my rules then I sometimes believed that I was not a good father to him. On the other hand, if I managed to keep all my rules then I would think I was a fairly good parent.

The point I am making is that your values are attached to many other things which control why you feel, do, say particular things throughout the duration of each day. They establish and hold your beliefs together. The rules you make last a lifetime.

A lot of things you hold as important and value were set in you at an unconscious level by other people, your childhood, and your environment. Your values were set in you by people and your environment; it is possible you are oblivious of many of your values. I know I was at the start.

I had a high value on the opinion that authority figures had of me. I valued their opinion and believed their judgement was always right. I created rules based on the values I had on authority figures such as trying to avoid talking to them so that they couldn't see any flaws or weaknesses in me.

It is remarkable how one type, the authority figures could have a lot of unconscious stuff linked to it. The more conscious you are about your beliefs, values and rules, the better equipped you are to assess them and alter them if they are no good to you anymore.

Ok, it's time to stop reading now. I want you to fetch your note book and a pen and make a list of the 20 most significant, meaningful and important things in your life to you. When you have finished the list, I want you to really look at those things which mean so much to you. These things are your values.

Now I want you to circle the values that you feel are empowering and are good for you.

Now look at what is left over, the ones you did not circle. Write down three of those beliefs which you have been working under as a result of the disempowering value. Next I want you to spot and recognise at least two rules that you set yourself for yourself to keep up the disempowering value. The last thing I want you to write down is what outcome you were hoping to achieve from the value that was disempowering. Then change it for a value that will give you the outcome you want.

For example, I valued the opinion of how authority figures perceived me which was a disempowering value.

What my aim was in valuing their opinion was actually to receive confirmation from them that I am a worthy human being. I had to alter my value at that point. To change disempowering values and beliefs into empowering values and beliefs is vital in overcoming stuttering. You should understand that assessing your values and beliefs needs to be done regularly; it's definitely not a one off thing.

It is important to be consciously aware of your current beliefs and values. Struggling to do that regularly can be off-putting but as you get used to it, it will become a lot easier. You'll be able to recognise those parts within yourself with ease. Each value and belief that you reveal, assess and alter will take you one step closer to overcoming stuttering. As you go through this process you will start to become aware of your speech improving.

How Fear, Anxiety & Stress Take Part in Stuttering

When I began analysing my stuttering patterns, months back, right at the beginning. I was always amazed at the fact that I was completely fluent when I was alone. It didn't make a difference whether I was talking to myself, if I was reading or if I was pretending to give a presentation, I was always absolutely fluent when I was alone. I was very interested by that because for this very reason I knew there was nothing physically wrong with my speech mechanism. It was working fine and I could prove that to myself over and over again.

Nevertheless, what had become very obvious to me after looking at my stuttering patterns is that there were constant things which were always there when I spoke in front of others, such as fear, stress and anxiety.

The reason was then very clear to me. I did not stutter when I was alone because there is no fear, stress and anxiety when I'm alone. This made me eager to do what I could to lessen the fear, stress and anxiety which were connected to speaking to authority figures. If I could do that then I could overcome my stuttering problem.

A communication problem doesn't automatically mean that you have a speech problem. The majority if not all of us who stutter are fluent when we are alone.

So what we need to work on now is trying to resolve our communication problems by looking at stress, fear and anxiety when speaking to others.

The things which I found useful and were effective for me to lower my stress, fear and anxiety were by increasing my fear, stress and anxiety threshold levels, observing myself as an outsider instead of taking part and understanding how the brain processed data and what my reality was.

One of the things that were very effective for me was to basically increase my tolerance threshold level of when stress, fear and anxiety would arise.

Everyone has different tolerance threshold levels. We all know someone who seems to go 'nuts' when little issues take place such as someone who suffers from road rage at a drop of a hat. On the other hand, I am sure we all know someone who will always seem to be calm and hardly ever seem to be troubled by anything. The difference between the two types of people is basically the person who goes 'nuts' has a low tolerance threshold level for when things go wrong, whereas the other person has a high tolerance level so they come across as being more in control of their lives.

You can notice the range of threshold levels in people who stutter too. A person who stutters regularly will have a very low tolerance threshold level and fear, stress and anxiety would arise more quickly at any sign of having to speak with others. Those of us who do not stutter much or stutter only in certain cases have a higher threshold level, which is why the fear, stress and anxiety do not come about until they reach that threshold level.

Increasing your threshold level is a very efficient way to reduce stuttering and if you can raise your threshold level enough you may notice that your stuttering problem goes away altogether.

There are quite a few ways to raise your threshold levels but what worked for me was firstly to make sure my mind stayed focused on what I wanted. Your brain is designed to carry out your orders. This means that your brain is on your side and it wants to give you what you wish for.

On the other hand though, your brain does not have the capability to differentiate between what you want and what you do not want based only on your words. It is only capable to take and use instructions from you based on what you think about and what you are focused on. Your brain does not have the ability to work out if what you are focusing on is what you wish for or not. This is why it is very important that you stop thinking about stuttering.

Another thing which was effective for me was to observe events which happened every day from an observer's point of view and not from a person point of view who's taking part.

Let me explain as it probably sounds confusing.

We take part in the events which come about in our everyday lives. We experience them, we undergo the emotions that are linked with them, we take part in forming the result and then we assess the events after they have finished. We all do this, everyday, all day, there's no doubt about that.

We are all observers; we go through life observing our inner and outer world. We just don't think of ourselves as observers because we are actively taking part in the events which happen in our lives. Nevertheless, if we move our thought process and just watch how we communicate with the world instead of having a reason then we can move into a neutral position, where we don't take sides.

This process is very interesting because as an observer you're not involved in judging the events or what the end result will be. As an observer, whatever happens will be fine with you. So if you were feeling nervous, fearful, panicky or anxious, as an observer you would just observe yourself feeling those emotions and you would be ok to feel like that. Observers do not interfere; they don't affect what they are observing or try to change it. They do not judge. Everything and anything that happens is all right with them because their only purpose is to observe.

This works in lowering stress, fear and anxiety because biologically, stress, fear and anxiety need to be fed by the right intentions and thoughts to survive. When you try to resist something, your mind has to focus on what you are resisting. If your mind is focused on what you are trying to resist then all the thought energy it needs to thrive and survive will be reaching it. If you are observing stress, fear and anxiety instead of participating then you are focusing on observing the behaviour not on resisting the behaviour. This is exactly why an observer is so powerful. You'll be surprised at how rapidly the stress, fear and anxiety just fade away. At least give it a go. It might be quite hard to begin with because you are not used to looking at your life from an observer's viewpoint. Just carry on practising, it will get easier.

I learnt over the years that we allocate meanings to people, the environment and events which makes our outer world and that we have total control over how we distinguish our world.

I began taking in everything I could find out on this subject because in this case that knowledge was going to be powerful.

It is only after studying so hard that I managed to gain the knowledge to recommend what I have to you so far in this chapter. Going through and assessing your current values and beliefs will lessen and ease stress, fear and anxiety automatically because you are altering your disempowering thought process for more empowering thoughts. I cannot state enough how important it is for you to understand the impact your thoughts have on the way your life turns out. It is necessary for anyone who is serious about overcoming stuttering.

Move Your Thoughts From Stuttering To Fluency

Move your thoughts from stuttering to fluency. Let me explain this through an example. If you frequently think about, or are anxious about, or are worried about stuttering then your brain only sees stuttering on your mind so it will make you stutter. If you frequently think the words 'I do not want to stutter' then your brain will still make you stutter because you are still focusing on stuttering. Your brain only sees stuttering, it doesn't see the fact that you do not want to stutter.

We all know that those who stutter are obsessed with thinking about it but if you can't think about it then what are you supposed to think about? The answer is easy. Think about fluency.

Think as much as you can about fluency, as much as you ever thought about stuttering. Think about all the times when you are fluent even if it is only when you are alone. How does it feel to be fluent? Can you picture it in your mind? Capture that picture and every time you begin to think about stuttering then stop and replace it with that picture of fluency. Think about fluency when you fall asleep. You've been living and breathing stuttering all your life, now it's time to live and breathe fluency.

When I realised how important it was not to think about stuttering, it was one of the most difficult parts of my journey because I had spent most of my life thinking about how to avoid stuttering. Moving my focus from stuttering to fluency was a regular battle at first.

I struggled so much and a lot of the time I really believed I could not do this. Then one day, everything changed, I was in total control at last. I was not thinking about stuttering at all, it had been replaced with fluency.

Whenever a stuttering thought entered my mind, I would replace it with the word 'fluency.' I actually felt calm and confident every time I said the word 'fluency', whether it was out loud to myself or in my head. The best thing was I stopped thinking about stuttering. To be honest, I haven't thought so much about stuttering for years until now whilst writing this book.

What you Should Expect on Your Journey to Overcome Stuttering

As you go through your personal journey to overcome stuttering you will be astonished at what you discover about yourself. Some of the emotions and feelings you will experience will be joy, eagerness, excitement, shock, doubt, discomfort, elation, disbelief, impatience, peace, annoyance and many more. It is vital that you make it ok to experience any emotion that comes along your way. Do not try to resist any of it. Let it happen and be determined to let it be ok.

When you experience a disempowering or negative emotion just recognise it, allow it and accept it, then observe it. Once you move into an observer's point of view it will decrease and then silently go away.

When you notice a positive emotion then enjoy that feeling.

In due course, you will eventually experience the past memories which you had forgotten as they come back into your awareness. You will also have thoughts which will come out of no where. They usually come when you least expect them like when you are driving the children to school or you're out to dinner with your wife. When those thoughts come you will know that you are that little bit closer to achieving fluency.

A Recap Of The Steps

On your journey to fluency you need to develop a firm belief that you can overcome stuttering. Stop wasting your time trying to work out who or what is to blame for your stuttering problem. Try to understand how the brain works and how thoughts affect the way your life turns out. Understand your current values and change them if you need to. Remove or increase your threshold levels for stress, fear and anxiety and move your thoughts from stuttering to fluency. If you do these things you'll be well on your way to overcoming stuttering.

Lets Talk!

In this chapter I will explore practical steps that stutterers can take to prevent stuttering. The complete holistic approach to curing your stutter involves both mental and physical training. In the previous chapter I talked about the importance of being mentally prepared; now I will discuss the practical everyday skills you can develop.

Opening your Mouth

People who stutter are always worried about getting stuck on a word (blocking) because the person they are trying to speak to will become aware that they have been blocked, which can cause awkwardness as well as humiliation.

To try to eliminate this blocking being so obvious, the person who stutters tends not to open their mouth wide enough and at times they do not open it at all. I used to try and say the word 'Podiatry' with a closed mouth and more often than not I would get stuck, which makes you wish that the earth would open up and swallow you.

At the time I would get stuck I really didn't think that just opening my mouth wider would make a difference. It now seems like the elephant in the room, as it's so obvious. If you open your mouth your voice box also opens which makes it easier to "breathe". If you look at fluent speaking celebrities they tend to have more movement of their mouth and jaw, it allows them to breathe easily which makes speech more fluent.

I would recommend you practice in front of a mirror and try and over emphasise your mouth opening, this is going to feel weird at first but trust me persevere with it. Then try and talk to a loved one with an emphasised open mouth, eventually you will get to a stage where you will train your brain to understand that it has to open your mouth to talk.

Emphasis

It is necessary that the key words in a sentence are emphasised. The key words are adjectives (describing words), people's names, places such as cities and countries. When we shout we do not stutter. Why is this? The answer is emphasis. This is why we have to apply emphasis into our speech. When you emphasise a word, it is not possible to stutter on that word unless you do not remember to breath or of course your mouth is closed.

I used to watch newsreaders and watch how they would emphasise certain words during a sentence. This concentration on emphasis inadvertently teaches you to breathe because as you emphasise a word you automatically take a breath. Try emphasising "football is a wonderful sport" I would emphasise football and wonderful which would allow for more fluent speaking. I also find that using my hands to emphasise certain words helps me to overcome a block. Body Language includes hand and arm gestures, facial expressions and any other body movement. This non-verbal communication serves 3 purposes, it illustrates and emphasises what you are saying when you talk. It makes talking more interesting, i.e. it will assist in keeping the person you are talking to attentive and it helps release nervous energy which can trigger stuttering.

Breathing

When we are born our breathing is naturally correct, babies can breathe, yell and scream with optimum effect because they use their lungs without conscious thought. As we grow older, stutterers can become lazy in their habits by only using the upper part of the lungs, taking a shallow breath instead of a normal one.

Let's examine the process of breathing in relation of talking. You breathe in to fill up your lungs capacity and then to start talking you let a small amount of air out and commence your first words. Some people can carry on talking until all the air is out of their lungs as with every single word that is spoken more precious breath is exhaled. A fluent person will breathe in between words but stutterers will carry on until they suffer from a block. The average person takes a breath every 6-7 words.

Most of those who stutter speak quicker than the fluent person on average, and when they reach that danger level when the air is running out of the lungs, they will tend to carry on talking rather than re-breathe, particularly when they are speaking fluently, they just don't want to stop. If they totally run out of breath, it will not be possible for them to speak. Let me give you an example, lets say a fluent person was to say "interest rates have fallen but the economy is in a downslide" A fluent person will take a breather after the word "fallen" a stutterer will typically try and get to the word "economy" before breathing.

I would actually advocate taking a breath every two words. This not only ensures that you do not stutter but also has a calming effect on you.

It's not only knowing where to breathe but how to breathe too, whenever you breathe directly through your nasal passages, the air that you breathe in is made pure and once it gets through to your lungs and goes out of your lips, it can then be optimised and leveraged in full. If you do this on a regular basis you will reduce your stuttering dramatically. Make every attempt to acquire a few purifying breaths through your nose before you begin talking. Fill up your lungs and breathe out directly through your nose. Always remember and keep in mind that when you breathe in you are breathing in the good and when you breathe out you are breathing out the bad.

This tends to be really simple and the payoff is immense! Also remember to stand tall, upright with good posture as it will enable easier breathing while talking.

Try this breathing exercise that will help you to learn how to use your stomach to help you breathe and therefore help cure your stutter. Lie down on your back. Put your hands on your stomach. As you breathe in, your hands should expand and rise with your stomach. When you exhale, your hand should return to the resting position.
Inhale and Exhale to the count of 5 (increase this number as you get better at it) with average lung capacity inhaling and exhaling to a slow count of 10 is good! Focus on your inhaling and exhaling, watching your hands rise and fall.

There are variations to this exercise you can also make a noise on inhaling - pucker your lips and suck the air in. Inhale through your nose; keep your mouth completely closed. Make noise on the exhaling or whistle as the air goes out. Put your hands behind your head, elbows out to the sides, this will expand your lungs even more!

Exchanging Words

When you stutter you tend to avoid certain words, it's only natural that you don't want to be humiliated in front of friends or family. So in my head I had "bad" and "good" words or sounds. Imagine having a conversation but you're picking the words that you're using carefully, not because they are more appropriate but because they are easier to say.

I would always ask for the wrong thing if it helped me avoid a word I couldn't say, but you get used to it. Eventually you do get what you want but not by asking for it straight out. I used to use the long hard way because I felt like I had no other choice. I thought it was the easiest way but now thinking back at it, I realise how much time I wasted.

By avoiding and substituting those words I found it helped me in the short term but made my stutter even worse in the long run. Every time you try to avoid a word, it becomes so much more difficult to say the next time round.

Slow Down

Those who stutter find it really hard to speak under pressure. When you are under pressure your voice box will automatically close up, not totally but with the same result as not opening your mouth wide enough. This stops a lot of our words to flow freely, which is why we have to speak slowly.

One of my friends who is into political activism gave an interview on television recently. Now he was pretty nervous at the time but when the lights came on her and the camera rolled he was perfectly fine. He normally speaks at 100mph; you can't get a word in when he's talking! But when he did the interview he was under pressure which caused him to really slow his speech down and breathe.

I was watching him talk but not listening to what he had to say but rather how he said it. It is vital that we speak slowly under pressure.

It's just like driving a car too fast, you might get a speed ticket or crash the car but either way you're going to be disappointed. Now conversely if you drive slower you will have a more comfortable journey and you will arrive more refreshed. That's just like talking, especially when we are under pressure. Pressure of talking to a certain person or in a certain environment makes us speed up our speech which causes a tightening of the voice box and hey presto, we stutter.

Just slowing down your speech will not prevent you from stuttering as you need to remember everything else about breathing, opening your mouth, emphasising words, etc but you can only do this if you give yourself time which is why you should slow down your speech.

Appetizer words

I call appetizer words the entry into a big word. For example if someone put me on the spot and asked me a question I used to get nervous and try and say the answer as soon as possible using the quickest route. So if I was asked what I would like to eat, I would reply steak. 9 times out of 10 I would get stuck on the letter "s" in steak. If I used appetizer words I would have said "I would like a steak."

This does several things, it slows down your speech but more importantly it helps you breathe so I would take a breath after "a" which would make saying the "s" in steak easier. It will also cause you to slow down.

Using the Telephone

For a number of people who stutter, the thought of using a telephone fills them with dread. However we can remove this anxiety by analyzing our behaviour. We do this by thinking about the advantages and disadvantages for those who stutter when using the telephone.

A disadvantage of using the telephone is that you cannot point to something saying "I would like that" or use your body language to convey a message.

But a huge advantage is that you cannot see the person so you do not have to worry about eye contact which can trigger anxiety. Also I find that use of hand gestures while I'm speaking on the telephone helps me not to stutter, I would often over exaggerate the hand gestures which is something I wouldn't do in a face to face conversation. Using the hands in this way helps expel nervous energy and also can aid in providing rhythm to the conversation. I will discuss the importance of rhythm a bit later on.

Also a very simple but such an effective method of helping you not to stutter on the telephone is to have a small piece of paper hanging on the wall next to the phone that says" breathe!" A gentle reminder will help you remember to breathe which allows you to speak fluently.

Job interviews

Everyone has to work for a living, unless you marry a rich footballer! However the thought of a job interview is such a mind numbing experience for most stutterers that it takes on an entity of its own. It is hard enough having to compete with 40 other people for one post but to have to overcome the fear of being a laughing stock just adds icing to the cake. I remember going for a job as a senior podiatrist when I was 21 years old, I didn't sleep for two nights before the interview. It was not because I wasn't prepared or qualified for the post but it was the fear that I would stutter in the interview. In my head it would be better if I didn't get the job rather than stutter in front of my peers and suffer the embarrassment that goes along with it.

At that particular time of my life I had very little control over my stutter and no one really to turn to. If I did approach my friends I would hear the classic line "just try and relax and you will be ok" In my head that was like someone holding a gun to my head and saying "relax things will be fine", I know that's a major jump from a job interview but the fear of the interview was that immense.

Over the years I have developed more control over my stutter but I can still impart some words of wisdom on the subject of the job interview. Stuttering can have a stigma attached to it, there are people who have stereotypical views that a stutterer will not be able to carry out their duties effectively or be able to mix with work colleagues in a social environment.

Generally employers are looking for an effective, productive, dependable and honest employee. An employer will ask varying questions in order to assess these qualities. The interviews will be structured so they can measure your capability, technical skills and test your judgment in your behavioural patterns.

Your stuttering will not stop you from showing your skills but there is a risk that the employer may have some preconceived stereotypical ideas about stutterers that you can address during the interview. There are various strategies you can employ to counter the perceived effect that your stuttering will have on the employer. Firstly do not mention your stuttering on your CV. When you speak about stuttering, speak about it in a positive manner and never in a negative way. You could say "due to my stuttering I have raised awareness of this issue in my local community".

You could also introduce yourself and your stuttering to the employer as "hello my name is .... And as you may have noticed I am a stutterer. I mention this because if I repeat or hesitate during talking it's not because I'm nervous!" This will instantly portray that you are confident. Or if you are not comfortable with introducing your stutter in such a forth right manner you could also mention "as you may have noticed I stutter, if you have any questions about stuttering please feel free to ask me." This action will show the employer that your stuttering has not had an effect on your self-confidence.

Most jobs emphasise that good verbal skills are essential but you can mention that it is also very important to be a good listener, formulate logical replies to queries and have excellent diplomatic skills. It's not the quantity of the words you can say in a minute it's the quality! Never let your stutter be a weakness but always portray it as a strength.

Obviously if you follow the advice in this book you will not need to even consider stuttering as a problem as you would have cured it, but if you do regress then you need to have these tools at hand.

Pausing

Pausing is a method that I've tried to employ over the years with varying success. Pausing can be done in many different ways. For example if the speaker gets stuck on a particular word you can pause for 2-3 second then silently mime the word and then re-attempt it. This pause has a calming effect on the speaker and allows them to overcome the word they were stuck on. For example, you can pause during a conversation if you have got stuck on a word as this will initiate you to breathe and will also have a psychologically calming effect on you. Your throat muscles will relax and anxiety will be reduced, in some cases you can also mentally prepare yourself for the next sentence. Pausing also insures that you do not talk quickly; many people who stutter try and finish a sentence off quickly due to the fear of stuttering. Another method is to deliberately pause between words for example after every 3rd word you pause for a second. These small pauses should not exceed a second and will encourage the speaker to breathe at the right moment.

Try saying the sentence below and pausing for a second at each comma:-

"Pausing, helps to relax, vocal cords, and, has, a, calming, effect, on, you"

I also found that pausing after the first block helps to prevent the domino effect of stuttering. This is when the fear of stuttering after the first block increases anxiety and vocal cord tension. This teaches the speaker to move on from actual or anticipitated further stuttering sounds.

You can practice this with a partner, friend or a loved one. Try to pause on every 3rd word to begin with and ask the person to raise their finger to prompt you to pause.

Try talking for 2 minutes about a random subject with pausing and 2 minutes without to see what affect it has on you. Pausing can take time to get used to and you may find it strange to begin with but it is worth persisting with. I used to record my own voice while using this pausing technique so that I could listen to how fluent I was. This would give me enormous encouragement so I would be more confident in using this technique out in the "real world". Eventually you will do it without noticing it.

You can also use pausing to teach a child to use the pausing technique. As I mentioned before my son also stutters and I have tried many different methods in trying to make him breathe in-between words. I recently used an abacus to teach him to pause in between words.

At first I got him to pause in between each word by moving a bead after each word, so I got him to say:

"I, love, Spiderman, because, he's, cool, and, I, love Harry, Potter".

After he got used to single word pausing I would ask him to pause after 2, 3, 4 words. It doesn't matter if he stuttered as I was rewarding him for pausing in between words by giving him encouragement.

You can also use the pausing method inside words. I'm not too keen on this method as it really interrupts your fluency but I find it quite hard to say "podiatrist", I would get stuck on the P, but if I say "Po...diatrist" I have broken the word up into two sounds with a pause in-between.

You can potentially do this with any sound you get stuck on but it may not be everybody's cup of tea (or coffee if you are that way inclined!).

Rhythm

Have you ever noticed that a person who stutters will not stutter while singing? That does not mean that all stutterers should walk around singing like they are permanently in the sound of music! But the variability of stuttering patterns is very interesting. Not all stutterers always stutter which can be confusing for the speaker and the listener. While singing we are effectively communicating in a rhythmic fashion, the speaker does not stutter as you are following the beat of the music.

This got me thinking, is there something I do while singing that I don't do while I'm talking. Well one of the main things I do is to breathe at the end of a line. A song, unless it's a fast hip hop song has regular breathing spaces. I also emphasised certain words more which helped complete them. For severe stutterers you could use this technique to teach your self breathing and talking in rhythm. For example, when sitting down place your hands on your knees and use them as drums. After every single word you can hit your knee to make the words come out more easily. You will find it easier to talk, this is not about permanently changing the way you talk but can be used as a tool to overcome troublesome words or sounds. As you progress with this technique you will no longer need to effectively create a rhythm as you could use your fingers without contact to create the rhythmic effect.

It is not only singing or talking in rhythm that produces this effect. It seems that singing and shouting are all forms of communication that are processed by the right side of the brain. This part of the brain deals with negative emotions such as depression, anxiety and more importantly for stutterers, fear. When we speak, we process information from our left side of our brain but research suggests that stutterers will use the right side of the brain more at times of stress and anxiety.

Some stutterers turn to hypnotherapy for help and recent research has developed a technique in which a patient is told to visualise the left side of their brain lighting up just as they are about to speak. This improves fluency of the stutterer; I have my doubts if it can be that simplistic as it may be a placebo effect or distraction technique. Nevertheless clinical trials have proven successful using this technique.

Caffeine

Caffeine is an addictive drug that affects the brains natural state, it stimulates it and has a similar effect to amphetamines but obviously not to the same degree. Caffeine also stimulates the production of dopamine. Research has suggested that stutterers have naturally high levels of dopamine which is a neurotransmitter; it makes you feel alert and motivated. Some studies have found that we have between 50-200% more dopamine in our brains compared to fluent people. Dopamine affects the basal ganglia of the brain which controls our speech mechanism.

So it makes sense that we don't drink anything that over stimulates dopamine levels, it's just like filling a car up too much with oil, its going to overflow and affect your exhaust fumes. This is the same with dopamine levels, the more higher the level the more it affects our speech.

Caffeine also blocks an adenosine receptors ability to slow down nerve cells in the brain which affects speech and also causes blood vessels in the brain to constrict.

I enjoy a cup of tea or cappuccino but I have reduced my consumption drastically and have noticed this has had a positive effect on my stuttering. The short term loss of alertness, renewed energy levels are insignificant when you start to talk fluently.

When stutterers say that they are having a good fluent day as opposed to a bad stuttering day it may be due to the levels of neurotransmitter i.e. dopamine. Dopamine levels can be affected by your diet. A high fat diet increase dopamine and research has actually suggested that a low protein diet would have a positive effect on your stuttering. I tried this but it didn't suit my lifestyle as I'm a gym fanatic and need protein for energy.

Just like with most things in life, caffeine is fine in moderation but I would recommend not consuming huge amounts.

Anti-Stuttering Medications

I would never take medication to control my stuttering, I haven't done it in all these years and I don't need to do it now. Not to mention the severe side effects that you can get from these medications. I sincerely believe that if you follow the advice in the chapters "it's all in your mind" coupled with the advice in the "lets talk" chapter; you will be able to cure your stuttering like me. However, I think it's important to mention stuttering medication just so that you can understand what health professionals are talking about when or if they ever attempt to try prescribe them to you.

Dopamine Antagonists

These are medication's that reduce dopamine activity, as discussed earlier this can increase the frequency of stuttering.

Examples include Haloperidol, Zyprexa and Risperdal. These can be effective in reducing the frequency of stuttering in low stress situations but patients can get severe side effects including increased anxiety, dizziness, hormonal side effects, rashes etc.

Dopamine Agonists

Dopamine Agonists increase dopamine levels, which should increase stuttering. Well that's what we thought but some doctors don't believe there is any medical evidence to support this theory. So medication such as Ritalin has been given to increase dopamine levels to control stuttering. This has side effects such as reduced appetite, headaches, increased paranoia, seizures and increased blood pressure.

Anti-depressants

Some stutterers can understandably suffer from severe depression which can cause them to seek professional help. The doctor may prescribe anti-depressants such as Prozac; these can increase dopamine levels which in turn increase the frequency of stuttering. So in a catch 22 situation as they make your depression worse.

Public Speaking

For too many people the notion of speaking in public has the effect of rendering one speechless. In the case of people that stutter it's a huge issue. Some studies show that many stutterers view public speaking as their number one fear.

We live in a society in which communication is vital and crucial to our everyday way of life and survival. So many professions and careers require us to address an audience of some kind and size at one time or another. Teachers, business people, retailers and journalists – just to name a few, all speak in public. Some circumstances may require a more formal delivery of information and may be more nerve wrecking than others which are more casual and generally presented to smaller audiences.

What many stutterers with a fear of public speaking do not realise is that whether at work, at home or at school, we all do speak in public on a daily basis at one level or another.

Fluent people and stutterers get nervous about public speaking. It's just that we are not nervous about the outcome of the speech where it didn't go down well but rather that we will suffer from a block which will cause us humiliation. The first thing to remember is that we have to do everything we can to be prepared for a speech. Such as becoming familiar with the place in which you will speak. Arrive early and walk around the room including the speaking area. Walk around where the audience will be seated. Walk from where you will be seated to the place where you will be speaking. Know your material well. Practice your speech or presentation and revise it until you can present it with ease. You can ease tension by doing exercises. Sit comfortably with your back straight. Breathe in slowly, hold your breath for 4 to 5 seconds, and then slowly exhale. To relax your facial muscles, open your mouth and eyes wide, and then close them tightly. The most important thing you have to do is visualise yourself making the speech and for it going very well. You need to focus on your material and the success you will have after making the speech and not on your stutter. You must not worry about your stutter as this will cause anxiety and lead to the very thing you don't want, remember the law of attraction! Use all the techniques in this chapter and you will be making public speeches in no time at all.

Improving Your Self-Confidence

What Is Self-Confidence?

What is self confidence? For those who stutter, having the self confidence to believe that you can speak fluently without embarrassing themselves would be a good start. Self confidence is a behaviour which is considered to be positive belief about yourself, where you can take control of your life and know what you want to do in it. Those people who are self confident recognise their capability to do something and then go on to do it. They do not rely on the consent of other people to verify their way of life.

It is enough for them to know their own potential and ability to do something, and have the nerve to do it no matter what others may say. This is why stutterers need to improve their self confidence and know their self-worth so that authority figures stop taking over their lives. Self confident people gain from the opportunities that arise by making the most of them.

The process of gaining self confidence begins from childhood, but an adult can still achieve self confidence through will power, sheer determination and with the support of family and friends. If a child is treated like they are abnormal because of their stuttering then this can have a huge impact on their lives which can leave them with a shattered self confidence through childhood right through to adulthood, perhaps even through their entire life.

Parental support and recognition has a part in a child's self confidence. People start to develop their confidence whilst growing up. An important role of the parent's is to put self confidence in their children. Parent's who are always putting their children down or are critical of them without recognising their strengths unintentionally reduce the development of their self confidence.

Whereas, parents who are always prepared to give support whilst encouraging their children to go forward in life will generally raise self confident children. Parents who make their children feel accepted and loved regardless of their faults will most probably encourage self confidence.

Even if a child stutters, the parents shouldn't put their children down. They need to be bought up like any other child.

There are parents who blame their children for their stuttering, this is the worst thing you can do. Children have their whole lives in front of them, just put yourself in their shoes now and again and see how harmful some of your words and methods can be even if you are not doing that intentionally.

How to Increase Your Self-Confidence

Being short of self confidence is not relative to a person's abilities.
Actually there are many very talented people out there but they do not have the self confidence to be able to show their abilities, like those who stutter because their speech stops them from reaching their full potential. Increasing your self confidence will give you the power to go forward and not let anything get in your way.

You don't want to be like the person in this example. Your group has to make a presentation to a client. It is an important time because it is a chance to get your boss to notice you. It could mean a raise or even a promotion if you could just gather the nerve to stand there in front of these people and present your pitch. The trouble is your nervousness over your stutter gets the better of you so you end up in the background. You're awestruck when a colleague makes a captivating presentation of your pitch. She stands there beaming with confidence!

You think to yourself "Why can't I muster up enough courage and control my stutter to present my own work to these people when I know all the ins and outs of this project?" You lack the self confidence it takes and your colleague has bucketsful of it and plus she doesn't have a speech impediment to deal with. Getting over issues which make stuttering worse and increasing your self confidence can leave a stutterer speaking fluently and not having to worry about their speech impediment.

If you want self confidence then you have to constantly do the things that will help you increase your self confidence. Recognise your strengths and weaknesses and get the most out of them. Make as much use of your strengths as you can.

This will help you increase your self confidence. Do not anticipate everything to be faultless; you are bound to make some mistakes on the way. No one is perfect, everyone makes mistakes, you learn from them and you move on. Maybe you have past experiences to do with stuttering which stop you from trying new things, maybe you've already given up but it's never too late. Just make the intention and go for it.

Recognise your abilities and what you have a flair for and make a note of them. Do not under-rate yourself. Try to identify every little thing you have done which has turned out very good.

Learning new skills can also help make you into a better person. Everyone feels better when they achieve things. Search for things which help to make you feel good about yourself.

Think about past achievements, things which you have taken part in, things you have won, things which you been successful at. Then focus on these things and take it from there. These things are your strengths, they will give you the confidence you need to do other things in your life. It doesn't matter what other people think of your stutter, the only thing that matters is what you think. That by itself will make a huge difference in your life. Having the right attitude gets you a long way.

Developing your self confidence is not easy or as straightforward as you may think especially if you do not think highly of yourself which a lot of stutterers don't. If you want to increase your self confidence then stay away from things and people that will dishearten you and stop you from gaining confidence.

Do not dwell on your failures or mistakes you have made in your past as that will make you feel unimportant. Being pessimistic and having a negative attitude will not improve your confidence. It is best to think about the positive things that you have done and use them as your motivation. With time, you'll start to believe in yourself more, you'll have increased faith in yourself and with a bit of luck, more confidence too.

What Is Bad For Your Self-Confidence?

Fear is one of the main causes of our low self confidence. Self confidence is usually described as the skill of a person to have confidence and believe in their abilities. When a person has great self confidence then that usually means they end up having great self esteem too.

Self-esteem is said to be the 'worth' that we can put on ourselves. It is measured in our own value as a person, according to our behaviour.

On top of this, it is also known as the respect and admiration in which we hold ourselves in based on our beliefs of what we are as a person. This affects the way we feel about ourselves a lot, as well as our lives, our relationships and it also determines sooner or later what we accomplish and how we achieve them. Those who stutter a lot do not tend to think very highly of themselves. This belief has to be changed if you want to live a full and happy life.

The development and expansion of our self confidence begins with examining ourselves.

The mind should be scrupulously checked so that when damaging and negative inclinations are found, weakness are removed and a right pattern of thought and behaviour are strongly set. Remember when you assessed your beliefs and values earlier in the book? This should have helped you have a more positive outlook on your stuttering.

Research has shown that fear is a person's enemy which holds them back in achieving their self confidence. Fear is also one of the causes which worsen your stuttering. This fear is like an illness that can be detected and recognised. It mainly comes about from a damaged mental pattern, where the mind is allowed to constantly dwell on hesitant thoughts, inadequacy and failure.

If you allow this to happen liberally, without trying to stop it, it will end up affecting more or less every part of your life and everything you do. You can't run away from your stuttering as you can't spend the rest of your life without speaking so why dwell on the past. Maybe things didn't go right in an important presentation or you embarrassed yourself in a speech. If you hold onto those thoughts then you'll always make those mistakes, you'll never set yourself free. The subconscious keeps memories of the past and in certain situations they come back to us. From today, start afresh. Erase all those bad moments and think about all the good ones you'll put in their place.

Fear from stuttering, for example, giving a public speech can be shown in many ways.

You can experience nervousness, hesitancy, shyness, apprehensiveness and even a need of 'self confidence'. There are many factors which add to a person's fear. When we feel unconnected, our fear increases. In reality, we do not fear the people and our environment which is familiar to us which is why we are nearly always perfectly fluent when it comes to speaking to family and friends. An unfamiliar environment and strange people bring about fear. Thinking about being put on the spot by a tricky question can stop stutterers meeting new people or attending social gatherings.

You have to fight the fear by developing your self confidence. You can do this by accentuating your strengths.

Concentrate on what it is you are able to achieve and praise yourself for your strength and your struggle rather than focusing on the result. You can also observe and practice how to handle situations, even negative ones. You should know when to stop when you catch yourself in a negative thought and change it into a positive one. Break that negative thought pattern. Knowing your own self-worth is also very important, learn to assess yourself. This way you won't be relying totally on the opinion of others and maybe then your fear of authority figures will disappear for good.

You have to remember that self confidence can be developed, it's not inherited and you can overcome fear because you have the faith in yourself to do so.

A Fear of Being Rejected

At one time or another, most of us have probably been haunted by a fear. It can be caused by our fear of living or even being alone. Depending too much on other people's views, low confidence and not being able to control our own lives. Fear of rejection is a state of mind which makes a person feel inadequate, powerless and insignificant. It stops a person from saying or doing things because of the fear that other people may not accept them or may dislike their words or behaviour. This is true for stutterers as they do not know how others will react to their stutter. People who come across someone who stutter for the first time may not know how to react either. Those who have low self confidence will be very sensitive when it comes to their stutter, they'll take people's reactions to heart.

This is the last thing you should do. You need to become thick skinned; if people have a problem with your stutter then it's their problem, not yours!

A person who worries about what others think of them can make their own life very miserable because they can no longer speak without worrying about what others think. The fear of rejection can paralyse a person and put him off from being productive or dynamic. A person's individuality is gone the instant they change themselves to be what others want them to be. These people have low self-worth. Young people who want to be accepted often crave for attention but they do not have enough of a foundation of self acceptance so they rely on their peers opinions about them.

This is damaging to a person's growth because no room is left for them to express themselves, there's only place for self denial and the thought of what others think of you.

A person who fears being rejected because of their stutter can be regarded as a person who behaves without confidence. A person who is not sure of themselves will tend to stop themselves from trying new things. Having such a lack of confidence will make a person unhappy and bitter at the end of the day.

There are stutterers who will eventually become depressed and no longer love life because of their stuttering. Some may be perplexed about their true identity because they've let their stuttering hold them back their whole life and now they regret it. A person could be lacking in self-esteem and self-worth.

A person who thinks it's more important what others think of him does not have much faith in himself to begin with. Being short of self-esteem could have been a result from feelings of rejection put in him by his family or even friends. Some people may feel they are treated differently because of their stutter, which may make them feel rejected. That could also be their reason for the lack of self-esteem and self-worth.

A person who fears rejection will eventually be rejected by the people he looks at to confirm his self-worth and the ones who love him dearly. A person who has a habit of worrying about what others think will soon find himself in a complicated cycle of rejection. His behaviour will keep the people he cares about alienated from him. He will never be able to be close with them and to him he will see it as rejection and then this vicious cycle will go on and on.

A Fear of Failing

Society has placed so much importance on success that failure has become a word which is generally avoided. Some people use positive thinking to keep failure at bay. This does help but it also makes a person start to believe that nothing can go wrong, as a result, creating a false sense of security. Failure can be very hard to handle but everyone fails one time or another in their lives. Nevertheless, it's not the fact that you have failed which is important, it is the way you have dealt with it and moved past it in life. This is an important thing to remember for a stutterer.

153

Don't let the thought of failing or not doing well because of your stuttering stop you from having a go.

A person can either let themselves be saddened and let down by their failure or they can use that failure to build up their willpower to move on in life. The important thing to remember is that the experience of failing was not for nothing because you learnt something from that failure. People who fear failure should know that the most successful people in the world have failed numerous times in their lives. What made the difference was how they learnt from their failure and how they used it to succeed in life. The true failures are those who fail once and refuse to try again in fear that they may fail again. There are many celebrities and powerful people out there who stutter, look at where they have got themselves too.
That shows that nothing is impossible, it just depends on how much you want it.

Not knowing when or if you will stutter can cause anxiety because of the fear of stuttering and failing to control it. Most often than not, this will end up with you stuttering big time. The more a person thinks about failing because of their stutter, the more he will end up coming to that conclusion every time he thinks about it. Without knowing it, the fear of failure has made a small problem into a more complex one.

Being scared of failing is normal. The way you deal with it is what makes the difference. The best thing to do when you are confronted with fear is to remember that it doesn't take long for things to change.

One minute you might be really down but the next you can pick yourself up and start again. Don't let your stutter hold you back, keep on going.

Everyone should accept that they are not perfect, no one is. Everyone has the right to fail so give yourself another chance, everything may change tomorrow, just give yourself a chance to fight. Don't give up just like that! You may suffer from a speech impediment but you have to remember that there are people out there who will be worse off than you and they are still managing to live their lives to the fullest that they can. Let that be an inspiration to you.

Make sure you have someone who can support you when things get hard so that you don't feel alone and unwanted.

At the lowest point of most successful people's lives, they turn to their family and friends. Other people rely on their dreams to get them through and make it to the top. However you deal with it, if you are determined to overcome stuttering and increase your self confidence then don't keep it bottled

up inside, it won't help. Talk about your
fears and get it out of your system.

Being Afraid of People

Fear is a powerful emotion which at
times is caused by being aware of a
particular situation where you always
stutter. It is in fact, a person's reaction to
a genuine or apparent situation that
they can't control. Sometimes a
person's fear serves as a protection
mechanism.

It is believed that fear is usually inherited,
like when a child who may inherit
certain biological qualities from his
parents.

These qualities can have an effect on
how a person's brain controls a person's
mood and how he reacts to things
which may cause fear. A person's
current fears will also depend on their

parent's behaviour especially on how careful they are or how they react to danger.

Fear can be categorised into many categories but the most common are phobia, panic and terror. Phobia is an irrational and overstated fear of a particular situation or object. You may have a phobia of public speaking. Panic is typically categorised by a hysterical, out of control reaction to a certain stimulus.

You may have a panic attack leading up to an important presentation. Terror is the biggest fear of all, generally causing a person to become immobilised. You may be in front of a huge crowd of people, ready to give a speech but as soon as you start to stutter you may just freeze and not be able to go on.

A person who has a fear of other people is called Anthropophobia and people who have fear in general or of society are called Sociophobia. A person who often feels anxiety or discomfort in the company of other people like many stutterers can have this phobia. People who have this phobia are still able to lead normal lives; they just tend to stay away from social events, like stutterers who tend to avoid mixing with people they don't know. It is similar to stage fright or being scared of performing in front of an audience.

People's whole lives tend to be based around their stuttering which leaves them missing out on so much.

A person who becomes anxious will have sweaty palms, feel butterflies in his stomach, experience a drying of the throat and mouth and may start to have a panic attack as well as an increased heart rate. Such fear can have severe effects on a person's family life and career. A person who is anxious, and who has no control over his fears, loses his freedom to act. Fear of people may be a part of a person's shyness or lack of confidence in meeting other people due to their stuttering. A person who lacks in self-esteem and stutters usually avoids meeting people because they feel that they are substandard to them.

A person who has no confidence in themselves might be scared of meeting people whom they assume are greater or more able than them.

There is an impression of normalcy in fearing other people. It is normal to fear people who have more power in their hands, or people who may have superiority over you. It is also normal to fear performing in front of an audience especially if you are not used to being the centre of attention or that you've had bad experiences in the past.

While most of these fears are normal, a person should not let these fears take over their personality. A person should recognise that they have these fears and should do things to conquer such fears. Or else, they will forever be harmed by their fears.

If you fear meeting people because of your stuttering, then talk to your family and friends as much as you can. The people who know that you stutter and won't judge you or treat you like you're abnormal. Talk about anything, it is important for you to learn to be relaxed when you speak no matter who you are talking to.

You can also begin to mingle with the people in your community because you will be more relaxed and at ease talking to them. Try to talk to at least one new person each day until you build up the habit of greeting people you come across in the streets. A simple good

morning is enough to help you increase
your self confidence. Take tiny little steps
and slowly try-out speaking with groups
of people.

Do not let your stuttering overwhelm
you. You may have fears about
stuttering but you have to remember
that other people are not exactly fear-
less. What is important is that you
recognise your fears and you do
something to defeat them.

Stand Up Straight

Stand out with self confidence. If you
feel confident with yourself and who
you are then people around you will
notice that. Even if your stutter bothers
you, try to not to let it show.

Body language says a lot about a
person, including their self confidence.

Self confidence can be shown in many ways; one of those is through body posture.

Body posture is the way a person carries themselves. It can be a starting point for making first impressions when you meet someone; it usually sets an image of the person in the eyes of another. Making good first impressions can be very beneficial. For example, in job interviews, most interviews end within seconds. Of course, the interview itself can take some time, but the outcome has been made seconds after the applicant enters the room. He is usually assessed through his gestures, body language and posture.

When a person stands tall, they portray an image of self confidence. Having a good posture is a fast and certain way of building a good impression. What is a correct posture?

It is a conscious effort to keep the body aligned against the body's centre of gravity. Being aware of it is very important. It is a posture where there is musculoskeletal balance. A person with poor posture can easily be noticed, they'll be the person who slouches, with shoulders drooping and head bowed down as if looking for something they've lost.

What can we do to be able to fix our posture? To begin with you must remember that just like everything else, having a right posture requires a conscious effort and commitment. To develop a good posture you need to make some changes to things you do regularly in your day to day life. It may seem very difficult but it is worth it, not only does it add to a person's self confidence, it's also good for you and will keep you fit and healthy.

Walk with Confidence

We all know that people walk all the time, but the thing is, most people are scared of walking. People would rather look down at the street than put their heads up and look at the people who are walking amongst them. Some people tend to look all over the place, at advertisements etc or even pretend to be using their phones. These are signs of poor self confidence which take part when walking.

So, how can a person's self confidence be portrayed in walking? Self confidence is a person's own view about themselves and their capabilities. Walking is one of the most basic human tasks and generally won't need a conscious effort; hence, walking takes the focus off the trendy clothes and equipment and says a lot about the person's personality. Walking shows a person's ability to carry themselves in any kind of situation. Being confident when you walk is a good place to start for people who stutter as you don't have to worry about speaking.

Walking faster can develop a person's self confidence in a number of ways. People who walk faster are seen as significant people. Walking a little faster would make an impression that, that person is busy and is involved in important tasks. It is all about creating a self-image for others to see even if on the inside you are worrying about the next time you stutter. When walking faster to communicate a message of self confidence, you must not overdo it to the point of panting and looking exasperated. It's just a matter of carrying a lively and comfortable self.

Leaving a good impression through walking is a different thing entirely from getting the real benefits of walking. Image building can be short-term, but the benefits a person gets from walking will last the duration of your life.

Walking briskly would compare to burning at least five calories per minute. If a person walks a mile, that person burns 20% less calories than if he had run. This may look unsatisfactory and may well encourage a person to run rather than walk but this should be taken in the perspective of everyday life.

People usually complain about having too little time to exercise, which is why walking to your destinations when you can is suggested.

When a person exercises on a regular basis, he will ultimately feel the benefits of exercising. He will feel more relaxed, his breathing will become better and his muscles stronger. Exercising also makes the mind stay sharp and quick. It may even help with stuttering. Walking, as a form of exercise, involves the whole body co-ordination and therefore, it gives what people might regard as a whole body exercise. Walking also makes the mind stay sharp because through walking, oxygen is delivered more efficiently to the brain, and blood flow improves. Perhaps this would explain why walking faster can boost someone's self confidence. More than building an image for other people to see, walking also makes a person feel better, as a result boosting his confidence. Taking these little steps will move you that little bit closer to increasing your confidence and overcoming your stuttering.

Walking as a form of exercise not only gives numerous benefits to a person's physical attributes, it also adds to a person's happiness since exercising would make a person release more endorphins which are "happy" hormones. So if you are having a bad day with your stuttering then add in a little exercise to help you feel better.

We have discussed the benefits of walking and how it improves a person's self confidence.

You have to walk properly to move towards your goal of improving your self confidence, to do this you must consciously try to increase your walking speed by at least 10% until a time that you can walk at increased speeds without too much conscious effort. Walking too fast will make a person look stressed and full of negative energy which you don't want. Make sure you hold your head up and maintain it at eye level instead of staring at the floor. This will produce opportunities to make eye contact with other people. It's a non-verbal method to say "hi, how are you?" so there's no stuttering involved.

Walking doesn't need much effort nevertheless; walking with confidence needs a lot of practice and dedication.

Walking can bring about several benefits in different levels to the person especially in terms of self confidence. Walking tall is being tall amongst all the challenges in a person's life.

Shake Hands to Improve your Self-Confidence

Body language portrays a person's self confidence. Shaking hands is a huge part of a person's body language. First impressions are based partly on how a person shakes hands. Handshakes are accepted as a form of greeting like they were hundreds of years ago too. It is also a non-verbal way of greeting someone so you don't have to worry about stuttering right at the start of meeting someone.

If you think about it, carrying out a proper handshake isn't very hard at all. They are quite simple and can be done with little or no effort at all. Anyhow, as I have mentioned above, handshakes are more than a straightforward gesture, they put a person's self confidence across to the other person. Handshakes can go awfully wrong because of nerves or even being excited where you can miss important opportunities, it may even leave you feeling awkward and uncomfortable.

So how is a proper handshake carried out? Firstly move towards the person whom you want to shake hands with, make eye contact with that person. Give that person a warm smile. Extend your right hand towards that person at a comfortable angle and when that person extends their hand, grasp it until the webs of the palms meet. Shake a few times then make an introduction or a greeting. Make sure to finish the handshake after 3 to 4 seconds.

When someone moves towards you and offers you a handshake, it is a polite thing to stand up before shaking their hand. If you are carrying something in the right hand which you cannot put down, shake their hand using the left hand. If both hands are engaged, a straightforward nod and apology can be used.

In a party, you must hold your drinks with the left hand, leaving the right hand somewhat available throughout the event for any introductions that need to be made.

Handshakes are exchanged in business deals, dates, meeting with old acquaintances, job interviews and social engagements. It is important for everyone to make the right impression especially someone who stutters who have the added speech impediment to deal with.

There are a few times when starting a handshake is not the ideal option. In the business world, when someone faces a very important person, it is better not to offer a handshake, especially if you have nothing important to say to that person. The other time is when both of your hands are carrying things which you cannot put down at that time.

A handshake is way more than a simple gesture. It is a simple gesture which builds relations and can leave an impression of a person. Practicing good handshaking can take a person to higher levels, in his career and even in building relationships.

Make Eye Contact to Improve Your Self-Confidence

To say that the eyes are the windows to the soul may sound like a cliché, but they are. The eyes are also the mirrors of our self confidence.

A person can easily weigh up another person's self confidence by using eye contact. People with low self confidence do not like making eye contact. They would rather look at the ground as if they were looking for something they've lost. For someone who stutters the best way to create the impression that you have good self confidence even if you haven't is to make proper eye contact.

The eyes are the first things which are noticed on the human face and they leave a long-lasting impression to the person who is looking. The eyes can make statements at a momentary look like no other part of the body can make.

Even without saying a word, the eyes can reveal a lot about someone. A person who is trying to conceal his unhappiness can never really act as if he is happy without people noticing it. The eyes can interpret thoughts and insecurities which are imprinted in the deepest holes of a person's soul.

The eyes also act as an indicator to a person's self confidence. The eyes play an immense part in making relationships, building careers and in portraying genuineness, in general.

Making eye contact can be the starting point for relationships. For example, if a man finds a girl he likes at a party or a bar, he would look at her when she was not looking, when the girl looks back, the man would attempt to hold his stare for a few seconds then he would turn away. He would repeat this set of moves a couple of times while increasing the time he looked back after every move. He would then make his move in the direction of the girl or back away for good. Why is that? In making eye contact, one can convey interest towards someone else. The man's stare should certainly get the message across to the girl. Once the move is completed, the reactions of the girl are evaluated. Making eye contact is a give and receive thing. A person not only has to express but he has to also listen to the response through his eyes.

Holding the eye contact for the right duration will set the move for introducing yourself. Holding eye contact too long can get someone accused of being a mental nutcase or a freak, while not holding it at all will send a message to the other person saying you are a shy person with a little self-esteem and a lot of insecurities. So if you are scared of going to talk to someone because of the thought of stuttering, when you start to talk use eye contact to make the initial contact, when you know the other person is interested then take it from there. That way you won't have to worry about stuttering and making a fool out of yourself when the other person isn't interested in knowing you.

Job Interviews

Interviews only last for a few seconds because more often than not, the decision will be made through the first impressions. Making eye contact with the interviewer will make him see that you are serious in getting the job. A nervous applicant will pass up eye contact because of fear. This is not a very good thing to do because interviews are carried out to assess a person's ability to handle pressure. Interviews are also meant to show someone's ability to express themselves and what other better way to immediately express your personality than through eye contact?

Speaking in Public

One of the main things that can make or break the deliverance of a presentation to an audience is eye contact. Eye contact helps take the fear away from the person who is speaking by getting the audience closer to him.

Stress is mainly a consequence of being with the unknown and uncontrollable. Eye contact gives the person who is speaking some reality which is the audience. It also helps in getting the audiences attention. A person in the audience likes to feel noticed and making eye contact with them makes them feel that the presentation is being delivered to them at a personal level.

Making eye contact is a vital tool in expressing yourself and getting responses from others.

People should not be frightened or feel uncomfortable in making eye contact as long as it is done in a considerate and proper way. Try to relax yourself as much as possible when delivering a presentation, smile back to your audience and if you stutter, try to let it go and continue. Remember the saying "the show must go on"? Well walking away from an unfinished presentation would be more embarrassing than stuttering through it. It takes a lot of guts to carry on in that situation and the majority of the audience will realise that and appreciate you more for it.

Change the Way You Talk About Yourself

To improve your self confidence, it is important to change the way you talk about yourself.

Self confidence is a person's own belief in themselves. It's the confidence you have in your own actions, beliefs and capabilities. Having self confidence is the answer towards a thriving and satisfying life. Self-talk can be described as that little voice inside a person's head which can either be useful or damaging to your self confidence. This inner voice is usually critical, gives remarks, or praises your performance and behaviour.

People tend to think differently when it comes to self-talk in relation to improving your self confidence. Some people link self-talk to one of the obstacles to get through to reach that confidence in yourself. This can be true for people who cannot get rid of the negativity in their heads.

This can become a vicious cycle where a person is continuously trapped in spiral where their self-esteem is going downhill. Another way is a way you learn at school. Self-talk is believed to be an important asset in developing self confidence. This time the inner voice can be seen as a mentor, a teacher, a friend or someone who gives you constructive criticism or comments.

You can make the most of self-talk towards developing a strong self confidence by listening to your inner voice. Recognise the inner voice in you and listen to what it is saying. Ask your inner voice questions concerning your thoughts on stuttering, the situations which brought about these thoughts and any other things which could have irritated the situation.

Remember you are doing this to build your self confidence, so try to be as truthful as possible; it's for your own good.

After you have identified your thoughts, it is time to consider them. What are these thoughts saying in general? What kind of attitude towards you is being projected by these thoughts? How have you reacted to these kinds of thoughts in the past? Have they been useful to me and helped me on my journey to achieve better self confidence?

Another important thing to consider is the way a person reacts to the thoughts that are being said by the inner voice. A person might think that negative thoughts are empowering and that they give them the push they need to accomplish their goals.

Negative thoughts and comments can be helpful in the short term; however, they do more damage than good in the long run. Negative thoughts put a general feeling of despair and uselessness, especially if a person fails more than once in a particular task. Looking at life in a positive way will help you towards building your self confidence. When a person stumbles, the inner voice should say "stand up, you can do it! Don't give up" rather than "you're pathetic, you can't talk without stuttering! You'll never be able to do this."

The tone of the inner voice is as significant as what it is saying. Negative tones should be controlled and be turned into positive ones.

You can make a huge difference with positive thoughts. Dealing with your inner voice can be an intimidating task. If it's difficult to talk to someone who won't listen, it's even harder to talk and listen to yourself as there can be no reasonable argument that can take place. Getting rid of the negative thoughts inside your head will give the positive thoughts some much needed space. It is all about changing the negative thoughts to make them positive. Our perception of the world is based on our views of the world. You increase your self confidence by feeling good about yourself. The inner voice should not have control of the body it is in, the person is the one who should have control over the inner voice.

Life is all about perception. You can never enjoy life if you observe it with a lot of pessimism. This is also true when looking at your own self.

Self confidence is linked to having true happiness. True happiness can only come from within a person's heart and believing in your self is the only way to attain happiness.

Have The Right Attitude. Say "I can" Instead of "I can't"

Have you ever noticed how we are never really quiet inside our minds? Whenever we are by ourselves, away from others, we can't stop ourselves from thinking. It just happens naturally. We take in everything from our environment and respond to it.

In prehistoric times, man would rely on his instincts to survive. This is known as the fight-flight response in which a person instantaneously chooses to fight and overcome his opponent or run away to survive. The body when perceiving a threat increases and opens up its supply and energizes the essential cells to prepare for a fight or a run. The body becomes more alert; the muscles get all the blood they need, which is when sugar and fat are burned rapidly.

In current times, the fight-flight response is still useful in a smaller capacity for situations against robbers, or fighting for a prize. Soldiers need this even more. For the regular person, the only violence they encounter is generally verbal or on television. Nevertheless, what most people don't realise is the violence and pain they impose upon themselves inside their own heads. Human beings are expected to interact with others to have a good life.

You can't escape from this and people cope in different ways to make a living by working alongside other people. However, sometimes fight-flight responses take over and spill over into areas of interaction that do not require an extreme response. This can be due to disorderly use of unconstructive strengthening techniques in childhood, a distressing experience, genetics, the environment, etc. In the average person, this spills over into everyday life. For example, being the person your peers joked about because of your stuttering, trying to ask a girl out on a date, or getting chewed up and spat out by the boss. These are the types of situations that, to most people, are the times of tremendous tension and anxiety.

The only way to conquer these awfully demanding situations is to train yourself to see it another way. A "Can Do" mind-set reflects this attitude. To make the most of life, people have to agree to living to the fullest.

Having a "can do" attitude shows that life to you is a Journey

People are expected to make mistakes, it's natural. If it does happen, why make a big deal about it? Acknowledge the mistake, and move on from it. Be grateful that you had the chance to learn something new.

Don't take life too seriously. Life when taken too seriously only makes the tense person more stressed. Laugh and have fun. Understand that nothing is perfect. Make the most of everyday and be happy. Be grateful for what you have in life, just like you'll be grateful when you overcome your stuttering.

The "can do" person knows exactly why he is here because he has taken the time to work out why. Whether that purpose is to teach belly dancing, or to be a top leader of a country, the "can do" person does it with two feet firmly on the ground and his eyes fixed on the future. Imagine your future where you are fluent and focus on it. It will be your reality if you really believe it will.

Set Yourself Goals

Are you one of those people who has just realised that life is passing you by and you haven't got long to make all your dreams come true? Don't let this happen to you. When you set goals use a timeline. Set yourself goals to help you gradually build your self confidence and focus on becoming fluent. When you set goals you have to keep going back to them and checking up on them. This is to set up the goal in your mind constantly. Eventually your mind won't need to be reminded about its goals. It'll set them for itself.

Your goal must have as much detail as possible. This is to cut the time it takes to think about what the goal is. It must answer the basic questions of Who, What, When, Where, Which and Why. The more detailed the goal, the more the person who set the goal will be able to imagine the outcome. A mental picture, an image helps hugely in the accomplishing of a desired goal. When you set goals, it must also be specific enough to show that you are making progress, for instance, if you had found it difficult to speak to strangers and used to avoid it but now you still find it difficult but you speak to them then you will know what you have achieved. Your goal must have a deadline. This is to stop you from putting it off. Give yourself enough time to build your confidence and if you haven't by the end of that time then consider why that is. What is holding you back?

Smile Even If You Have No Reason to Smile

Have you ever tried to smile and think a negative thought at the same time? It sounds impossible doesn't it?

Usually the outcome will be that one of the feelings will win out. It might make you feel better because you smiled or you will ultimately feel bad and mope, this is a significant fact in human psychology. Humans cannot in fact hold their attention on more than one thought at a time. This is the answer to mastering yourself in this life.

The human is the only organism so far which is known to be aware of its own existence. It is possible to use the will to make a choice on how a person reacts in a situation.

Smile even if there is no reason to smile. It will promote a sense of positivism that clears out negative thoughts. On the other hand, if you frown you may find yourself too stern to even let people near you.

Our thoughts are like fluid, they are always moving from one state to another. The test is to manage to keep them where you want them. Think about fluency and forget about stuttering.

Use breathing methods to help you clear your mind and relax. A sense of detachment and awareness of your state is the key to dealing with unstable emotions.

The effect of breathing is that focussing on the breath is a supply of calmness and control which is very much so needed when a person needs a sense of control. Breathing deeply and focussing on it also loosens the hold on the sense of self. It gives the body more oxygen to fight the effects of stress and tension.

Express How Great You Are Daily

All sorts of people from anywhere in the world uses affirmations to keep themselves going. Bank managers, teachers, psychologists, students, and even politicians use affirmations. This is because affirmations are a positive way of reminding themselves of their choices and their goals.

Affirmations are clear as declarations of the belief of a reality or truth of a thing. This is one of the basics of self confidence and the way you can deal with the world.

There are times when we lose track of ourselves. It happens at work, at home when taking care of the needs of your family, or meeting your targets in your workout at the gym. We have no idea why we are doing anything. Most people go through life without setting goals.

People with goals are more confident of themselves because they measure themselves against a target. This lets them know where they actually stand against the goals they have set. It can be understandable that people lose their way after they set the goals. This may be because they do not have the device to continuously affirm their actions. Or there was no system set up to affirm the goals they have set, which reminds them why they are working so long and hard for. This is where those little pieces of paper that I asked to put around your house about stuttering come in useful. They will remind you what you are doing this for and what you want to achieve at the end of it. Remember to always keep fluency on the mind; it'll keep you on track.

When you forget goals, a lot of time is wasted. With time a person loses his self esteem, his confidence, and ends up giving up. This is why it is important to uphold a high self-confident attitude that does not disappear from reality. The role affirmation plays on upholding self confidence is in the area of autosuggestion.

Autosuggestion is a statement of an intention or a goal which is repeated over and over again until the mind of the person accepts the statement as the truth. This type of affirmation is looked at positively and it combines a person's funds and effort towards the attainment of the goals.

It is also a way of reaching the subconscious and getting it to help you achieve your goals. It is a type of self-hypnosis; generally it comes with a forceful image with the statement. The person repeatedly tries to live through the moment as if it had already happened.

It seems that humans are fairly good at mentally programming themselves to accomplish a specific goal. People who are into sports know that this works, they visualise winning games and it happens. It has worked for many athletes.

Nevertheless, a conflicting effect can also take place. A person can repeatedly place himself in a place where negative thoughts continually attack the mind into compliance.

The brain makes out no difference between a positive suggestion and a negative suggestion. For that reason the wording of the affirmation has to be very important. It is always better to affirm a statement in a positive sense instead of the negative one because the mind does not hear any negative comments. For example, if a person wants to stop stuttering, his statement should not be "I will not stutter." The mind can only take in and accept it as "I will stutter." It would be better to say, "I will speak fluently."

The more positive the affirmation is the more powerful the effect of the affirmation will be. Affirmations must be fixed everyday. It should the first thing you do when you wake up, before you begin work and before you go to sleep. This is how you programme the mind for achievement.

Visualisation is carried out by seeing a future occasion in as much detail as you can, for example, imagine yourself giving a speech and being perfectly fluent. What would that feel like? The aim is to create a forceful vision that the mind will willingly accept as truth. If you do it correctly, the mind will work subconsciously towards the completion of that aspiration.

The mind is a very influential tool for victory. It is like a sponge, you must be careful what you or others put in it. Everything gets absorbed in. Use affirmations and visualisations to clean up your mind too. Nothing happens effortlessly. Nevertheless, try some of the ideas I've outlined here and in no time your self confidence will rocket! You can do it!

Stress

People's voices change under stress, even fluent people can produce a degree of dysfluency when under stress, and all stutterers know that severe stress can induce a block. As mentioned previously stutterers can talk fluently when they are relaxed and no one is present or they are in certain company. This is when stuttering is completely different to other medical conditions, have you ever heard of a deaf person that is only deaf around certain people!

All our brains are capable of fluent speech as we all have the mechanisms that can produce fluent speech. Like wise we all can produce stuttering sounds. Our brains select one or the other depending on the environment, for example if you are talking to a partner/ spouse, you may have reduced frequency of stuttering but you may stutter when ordering food at your local restaurant. Even if you have been to the restaurant on many occasions the environment is still not as safe and secure as speaking to your better half. Therefore your brain handles stressful situations by triggering it to produce a stutter. The subconscious choices we make to select what type of speech motor programmes will be activated can be altered. You can respond to stress with fluent speech if you can recognise the triggers and have options available to you. So much so in fact, it can be to the point where you can be more fluent than a non stutterer under pressure.

When you're stressed your heart rate increases which is why stress is linked to heart conditions.

Also when a person experiences stress, the brain responds by initiating 1,400 different responses including the dumping of a variety of chemicals in to our blood stream. Stress is not just a psychological factor as it also has physiological implications. Forty-three percent of all adults suffer adverse health effects from stress and an amazing 75% to 90% of all doctor's home visits are for stress-related ailments and complaints.

So you would think that when we stutter we are always stressed, think again. Systolic blood pressure (pressure in your arteries when your heart is forcing blood through them) is actually reduced by stuttering which will be bemusing to most stutterers. If you actually think about the sequence of events when we stutter then it makes sense.

We usually start off a conversation with a block or dysfluency which causes a huge amount of stress but as we begin to talk fluently there is a release of stress. We then suffer from another dysfluency which causes stress levels to rise but as we approach the end of the conversation this is when we are at our most fluent, your systolic blood pressure will peak at the beginning of the conversation and then gradually decreases as the conversation nears an end.

Stuttering reduces your stress levels for a few seconds as you manage to talk fluently but then as you suffer a dysfluency you end up back into the cycle of increased followed by a decrease of stress. That obviously has huge implications on your health as this yo-yo effect on your blood pressure is not good for your long term health.

The person listening to your dysfluent speech may also be stressed which in turn increases the stutterers stress levels.

Some speech therapists advocate using a distraction technique to help you cope with the stress levels and thereby reducing the frequency of stuttering. Such as concentrating on something else while talking, like the background or counting something in your head. However as most stutterers will tell you that it is hard enough concentrating on talking yet alone doing two things at once, people that know me will tell you, I find it hard enough concentrating on one thing for long enough! So this technique may reduce your overall stress but will increase your stuttering.

Types of Stress

There are many different types of stress, some produce stuttering while others can actually decrease stuttering in the short term. Have you ever been in a situation when your adrenaline was running through your body at a speed of knots? Some people can suddenly start talking fluently and clearly as the adrenaline is rushing through them. This is due to the adrenaline competing with the dopamine which inhibits dopamine production and reduces stuttering, the downside to this is that when the adrenaline reduces your stuttering increases.

I can have two completely different responses to an adrenaline rush, I remember once one of my friends had a severe asthma attack and I had to go and call the ambulance, I suffered a huge block and found it really hard to complete the sentence. On another occasion I almost got into a road rage fight which ended applicably which is good as the guy was huge! But I remember feeling an adrenaline rush and being as fluent as I've ever been. So your brains response to adrenaline may vary depending on the situation and the person.

Stress that is induced by physical exercise or physical pain may increase your stuttering unless you have programmed your breathing to relax your vocal cords.

Stress can also be increased when talking to someone that is not giving you their full attention. I have a friend who I call Woody Allen!

He's so hyperactive that he would not follow your conversation and jump to other topics like a grass hoper; he can cause my stuttering to increase. This type of stress is called cognitive dissonance. This is the feeling of uncomfortable tension which comes from holding two conflicting thoughts in the mind at the same time. Dissonance increases with the importance of the conversation you're having and the impact of the decision, along with the difficulty of reversing it. Discomfort about making the wrong choice of car is bigger than when choosing a lamp.

So in certain circumstances when you have two opposing views in your head and you're trying to communicate this to another person you may stutter.

Stress can also be caused by time pressure. Asking a stutterer to talk quickly will inevitably produce pressure which can result in stuttering. Or if you are trying to rush somewhere for a meeting and you're running late, the time pressure will produce stress which can increase dysfluency.

Another interesting observation is the type and atmosphere of the conversation. For example if you are talking in a serious manner your dysfluency may increase as apposed to talking in a more casual relaxed way.

The formal conversation also has different layers, if for example it was a formal conversation that was going to produce an outcome that you were expecting then it would produce a different response to a formal conversation in which you were expecting a negative response.

For example, if you're asking your boss for extra holidays but what you are expecting to hear may cause an increase in stuttering. Also if you're asking an attractive stranger for a date, that can cause more stuttering than asking a friend out on a date.

When you stutter the listener thinks you're stressed and their response may be to dominate the situation. Some stutterers will try and use the fact that they can talk fluently when having a casual conversation to their advantage. So even if they are having a conversation about a serious topic like asking for more holidays they may approach it in a causal laid back fashion. This is not always a good idea as the person may not think that you're serious about the topic and in certain circumstances such as paying your condolences to a family, it would be highly inappropriate.

I would recommend you prepare what you are going to say and if you are anticipating objections then you have the answers to them. Talk slowly, open your mouth, relax your vocals cords and think positively and use the techniques in the previous chapters to talk confidently about the subject you wish to address.

Speech Patterns and Stress

We tend to mirror each others speech patterns, for example if someone is shouting at you then you tend to shout back and if someone is angry with you this normally elicits an emotional response which culminates in an angry confrontation. Similarly if someone is talking very quickly you feel as though you need to also talk quickly to keep the flow of the conversation. These types of speech patterns will have a detrimental effect on your stuttering. So I would recommend you always do the opposite to what the person is doing. If someone is talking quickly then make a conscious effort to slow down your speech. Stuttering can also increase if you have a fear of being humiliated or embarrassed. If you are talking to someone and you are unsure of the response or if you have said something silly, your stuttering make increase. The easiest way to combat this is to acknowledge your embarrassment and try telling a quick one line joke for example" I think I'm going to take my foot out of my mouth now!" That always elicits a smile from the listener which will help in reducing the overall stress levels. If someone is angry with you, remain calm and make a conscious effort to talk more quietly, this will help you get your point across in a more controlled and fluent manner.

Stress can cause us to react irrationally rather than rationally to any given circumstance. If we can recognise the type of stress we are under then we can control our stress levels and thereby reduce stuttering. Moving away from an emotional or shameful stress response to a more measured stress response will enable you to have greater control over your stress pattern and ultimately reduce your stuttering. Always ask yourself when you are stuttering, how am I feeling right now? Then have a mental tennis match in your head and come to a rational response remembering to keep calm.

Psychology of Fear

There is a name for every type of fear. Are you scared of travelling? You have siderodromo. Are you scared of beards? You have pogonophobia. You can even be scared of fear itself phobophbia!

Humans are obsessed about being scared of something or the other and in most cases it's an illogical fear. Most people think that they are scared of either snakes or spiders. Even a chimpanzee starts to scream when they see a snake. The reason why humans fear snakes and spiders is because of our natural instinct that they can be venomous, which will have a negative effect on our health.

However, this is an irrational fear as in this day and age in most cities, they would be completely harmless. Unless you're living out in Africa or rural Australia, they simply do not pose the threat that we perceive in our minds. We should be more afraid of speeding cars, global warming, electrical failures, not snakes and spiders which are not even natural to our environment.

Hand on heart I used to be terrified of mice, now I don't know who would be more terrified the mouse or me! This was a fear I addressed long ago with my other fears about stuttering. I felt as though I needed to remove fear of all irrational things from my head. Even if logically I know that the mouse cannot hurt me but my psyche told me it was dangerous. This is the same as talking to certain people logically you know this person has no power over you yet your stress levels increase and you stutter.

What if I told you that now I look at a mouse as if it was a fork or a knife? I then wouldn't associate danger with the mouse and I have lost all fear of it. You can remove fear when you condition yourself to understand the type of fear and your response to it. Is there a person that you stutter around more than others?

Now I want you to imagine that person as an innate object that has no emotion and more importantly no power over you and see how it affects your fluency.

Fear and Stress

There are certain circumstances when you genuinely have a fear about the situation and your stuttering just compounds the fear. For example, speaking to an attractive person for the first time will make your heart skip a beat. Giving a speech at a wedding can be the most fearful situation, having friends and relatives watching you attempt to talk can make anyone nervous.

Stutterers combat this by avoiding certain circumstances so we may not leave a voicemail or ask for a date. Using this book you can combat all those fears by using the techniques set out in "it's all in your mind", "let's talk" and this chapter so you can accomplish what you have been scared of doing. Different things work well for different people so make a list of the advice in this book and find the areas you find most appealing to you and start using the techniques.

The only way to overcome your stuttering is taking the theories you have learnt and using them in a practical way. Make a telephone call to a friend you haven't spoken to for some time, order pizza at the local takeaway or go and ask for directions. You now have an array of powerful tools you can use so what is there to be scared about?
You are no longer going into your "fluent battles" empty handed and unprepared. All stutterers have a mental list of feared speaking situations they would avoid, mine was talking to strangers. I would always suffer a block when asking for directions. So after I had learnt the knowledge in this book, I went out of my way to speak to strangers. As you tackle your inner fluency demons you will remove the power they had over you and find it an altogether liberating experience.

After you have conquered these demons related to stuttering it's time to do what even fluent people would be nervous doing. Such as asking to speak at a family get together or even doing a toast at a dinner. You need to exceed your boundaries so you remove the very essence of your stuttering fear in you.

The listener

We often underestimate the effect stuttering can have on the listener. Stuttering is not as common as athletes foot (sorry had to mention a foot condition as I'm a podiatrist!). Also it's not something you can conceal as it will become apparent as soon as you start talking. The listener may think that you are nervous or even mentally deficient depending on their knowledge of stuttering.

Some listener's think that you must not be telling the truth which is why you would stutter. I remember an incident in my 20's when a police officer stopped my car and started to ask me some basic questions like what's your name, where do you live. As I had no control over my stutter and saw him as an authority figure, I had a severe block. This made him think that I was lying; he even asked me if I was nervous because I was lying! This increased my stress levels even more and my stuttering increased. What a vicious circle!

Generally listeners can get stressed or impatient by listening to a stutterer and will communicate this through their body language. This wil increase the stress of the whole conversation. If you do not have complete control over your stutter then tell the listener that you stutter and you are using techniques you learnt in a book to help you, Make a joke to break the ice, this is especially useful when giving a presentation.

Your life is in your hands

Stutterers try to avoid circumstances that can cause them to stutter. Some may even turn down promotions at work or jobs that involve talking to people or answering the telephone. Even if you use the advice in this book and recover from stuttering you may still believe that you still cannot talk as fluently as a fluent person. You may even describe yourself as a shy person. You need to change your mental outlook completely and start by doing the opposite of what you have been doing for so many years. Describe yourself as confident and apply for jobs you would not have even thought about applying for before. Make a positive intention that you will change your lifestyle as you no longer fear stuttering.

Relaxation and Guided Imagery steps

Meditation and Guided Imagery are techniques that use the natural power of the mind to reduce the stress caused by your stuttering. Einstein estimated that we only use 10% of our brains. In practicing Meditation and Guided Imagery, we have access to the other 90%. Since thoughts are one of the most powerful possessions we can have.

How it Works

Meditation and Guided Imagery work because the Physical Universe is energy; this energy is vibrating at different speeds. Energy is magnetic causing similar thoughts to attract other similar thoughts. What we dwell on is what we will attract. Thoughts and ideas are high vibrating forms of energy and are very powerful.

To be able to practise the exercise, I would recommend you ask someone who you trust to help you in recording the steps on a tape or CD, which you are able to listen to in private. It would be ideal to ask someone who you do not have emotional attachment with as it helps with being objective when dealing with your emotions. The exercise lasts approximately 20-30 minutes. Before you record this, you need to establish and inform the person of a place where you feel happy, relaxed and yourself. This could be at work, with friends, somewhere where you are comfortable and feel yourself. When instructed to go to a place where you feel happiest, the person recording the exercise must refer to this place where you feel this way.

Close your eyes.
I am going to start with counting from one to twenty, whilst I begin to do this, take in a deep breath and breathe out. Continue with the breathing pattern of inhaling and exhaling.

1
Pause
2

As you continue to breathe in this way, I would like to you to focus …….. (This is where they state your 'happy place') You know this place very well, this is where you feel good about yourself, you feel good, you feel like yourself and happy, strong, valued.

Pause
Just inhale and exhale
Pause
6

Whilst you are breathing like this, I want you to imagine on each out breath, you are breathing out feelings of anger, frustration, stress, anxiety, any feelings of depression…just let it all come out on your out breath.

9

As we are moving closer to 20, I would like you to carry on breathing the way you are right now, just to inhale and exhale.

Pause
10

Again think about ...... (Refer to the 'happy place' and describe it, the surrounding, environment, whatever it is that makes you feel good and calm)

12

Inhale and exhale

13

On each in breath, imagine you are revitalising the cells in your body, giving yourself oxygen, life and more energy...every time you inhale you are giving yourself more energy, replacing those energy fuels that have been depleted. Again when you breathe out you are breathing out stress, anger, frustration caused by your stuttering.

Pause
14
Just inhale and exhale
15

Again as we are moving closer to 20, I would like you to really concentrate on ....(your 'happy place') where you feel good, perhaps there is something distinctive, like the atmosphere, your surroundings, doing things you like, and how good you feel...strong

16
Inhale, then exhale
17

As you're inhaling you are becoming revitalised, when you are breathing out, you are breathing out negativity, stress.... It is all leaving your mind and body

19
Just one more step....just carry on to inhale and exhale
20

Excellent, just carry on inhaling and exhaling, you are doing very well
Now using your imagination, I would like you to imagine.......(a 'happy place') and in front of you there is a blank television, DVD and remote control, when you can see this nod your head to let me know.

Good

In a moment I am going to ask you to press play and see a form of yourself in the ....(happy place) on the television where you feel relaxed, calm, balanced, you feel really good about yourself, full of life, full of energy.........In a moment I am going to ask you to press play and see a form of yourself in the ....(happy place), relaxed calm, balanced, feel really good about yourself, motivated, strong, full of energy, full of life, full of enthusiasm, you can see how well you are doing.....
When I would like you to watch this film I would like you to watch it at a normal pace, so you just press play and you are going to watch this powerful image of

you, and when you have finished watching yourself, nod your head.............Just imagine pressing play, doing your thing, doing what you enjoy, what makes you feel good. When you have done watching the film let me know.

Good, very very good...........Just need to remind you that you can revisit this place, this frame of the film anytime you like.

Using your imagination again, I would like you to imagine floating up and above yourself, and you are now able to look down at yourself, sitting in front of the television, DVD and remote control. When you have achieved this, nod your head to let me know.

Pause for about 15 seconds

Good, excellent, you are doing very very well.

Now what I would like you to do is to recall an experience, it could be any experience you have had, recently or in the past, where you have felt really down about yourself due to your stuttering, low, depressed, angry, frustrated, low of energy, difficulty sleeping, difficulties with concentration...just angry with yourself for doing and feeling certain things, anything at anytime....I would like you to choose one particular occasion...
Use your imagination now.
I would like you to imagine looking down at yourself, and you are going to see yourself going backwards from the end of the experience all the way to the beginning before it had occurred.....so just imagine looking down at yourself pressing play and rewind, you are going to go back in reverse order, fast, to the beginning, once you have achieved this, nod your head to let me know.

Pause.......That's good, very very good

Everything you just saw on the screen looking down at yourself, now I would like you to imagine pressing play and forward, you are going to see the same experience but in fast forward motion, from the beginning all the way to the end as fast as you can.....again once you have achieved this, nod your head to let me know.

Pause...............Excellent. Now I would like you to think about......(happy place) where you were in a happy, positive environment... this is a good place, you are happy, valued, you value yourself and you feel good about yourself. You are relaxed, balanced and calm. Whilst you are thinking about your special place, I'm going to let you know, that after this exercise, tomorrow and subsequent days to come, you are going to feel balanced again, not only balanced you will have more energy, more focus, your memory is a lot sharper, and importantly you are able to sleep at night too.

Pause.

Again I would like you to recall anything, just to make sure that it will not impact you again, recently or in the past when you have felt angry, frustrated, depressed, down, very emotional and tearful...this could be at anytime, I would like you to select one particular time...again I would like you to visualise looking down upon yourself, and you are going to watch yourself press play and rewind, and you are going to go backwards through the experience in reverse order fast.....once you have achieved this nod your head to let me know.

Pause.....that's excellent....again using your imagination, I would like you to imagine looking down at yourself again, and you will watch yourself press play and forward.......You are now going to see the same experience in fast forward motion.........Again when you have

225

finished doing this, nod your head to let me know.

Pause......That's excellent, you are doing very well.

I would like you to think about.........(happy place) again, a relaxed environment, a very good atmosphere for you...........Just going to let you know, when you finish this exercise, all those strong emotions you had before the exercise will be gone. You are going to feel relaxed, calm, balanced and stronger. You will notice tomorrow after a good night's sleep, you will have more energy and be more focused again.

Pause

I want you to also recall, where you may go back some years, and again it doesn't matter which occasion you choose, the experience of frustration, self hatred, anxiety, that upsets you.....it doesn't matter which occasion you choose, I would like you to recall this specific time when one of the events happened, and again we are going to do this very quickly, to recall the experience, by pressing play and rewind, going back as fast as possible to the beginning...once you have achieved this nod your head to let me know.

Pause

Good, very very good...........Everything that you have just seen on the screen, I would like you to look down at yourself, this time I would like you to press play and forward. You are going to go through the same experience in fast forward motion....Again when you have reached the end nod your head to let me know.

Pause

Very very good......... I would like you to recall the.......... (Happy place) again, all those emotions, of anger, stress depression, traumatised memories have been neutralised. You are now free from them, when you finish the exercise you will feel some weight as been lifted off your shoulders. You feel calmer, relaxed and more balanced within yourself, tomorrow you will have more energy, and more focus to do the things you want to do.

Pause.

I would like you to imagine now, an image of you floating back into yourself, and what you can see in front of yourself is a television, DVD and remote control. When you have achieved this nod you head to let me know.

-
You are doing very well...........Now you are going to watch a short film of yourself set in the future, this is not very far in the future, it is in the near future. I'm going to let you know what is on the film. The film that you are about to watch is you in the future where you are calm, you're relaxed, no depression, no anxiety, no anger. More importantly

when you watch this film, you will notice how confident you are, in yourself, in your capabilities. You are a smart, intelligent person and you will notice how well you are doing. When you are at work, with friends, you are a lot more sociable, balanced in your mind and you are focused on your future. It is a very powerful Image of you. I want you now to imagine pressing play and you are going to watch yourself press play and watch yourself relaxed, calm, balanced, sociable, intelligent, focused and strong....When you have finished watching the film at normal speed, nod your head to let me know.

Pause

That's good, very very good..........Using your imagination again for the last part of the exercise, I would like you to imagine an image of you floating out of yourself and into the screen, and you are becoming a part of the film. You are balanced, relaxed, calm, together, strong, and focused, you have lots of energy, and you are sociable, smart

229

academically. So just imagine floating out of yourself and you are watching your image float into the screen and become a part of the film. When you have achieved this, then nod your head to let me know.

Pause

That's excellent, you're doing really well............I am just going to let you know that this is your future, and when I am counting back from 20, these are steps to your new future. Your future is bright, you have everything going for yourself, you are well, intelligent, you are very good at what you do, and you are going to learn how confident you can be, and how good you can feel about yourself. I am going to be counting backwards from 20 to 1, these are steps towards your new future, and each time when I am counting back, I would like you to focus on your breathing again, just to inhale and then exhale.

20
Pause

19

Pause

18, 17

Pause

16

Pause

15, 14

Pause

12, 11

All the energy you need is being
restored

10, 9

We have passed the half way stage
now

8, 7

6

Pause

5, 4, 3

3, 2

Pause

And 1...... In your own time after about
5 or 7 seconds you are able to open
your eyes.

Bullying

Bullying is a serious problem for stutterers not only at school but also at the work place. The bullying can be persistent and leave emotional scars that can affect all parts of your life for many years to come. Research carried out by Child line has discovered that more than half of the 953 pupils questioned have been bullied at primary and secondary school. Research carried out by the British Psychological society specifically on adults that stuttered found that an astonishing 83% have suffered bullying at school which ranged from name calling, threats, rumour spreading and physical aggression.

I was constantly bullied when I was in secondary school which would often end in physical violence. I remember the feeling of being alone and not having anyone to turn to. A child that stutters may not know that it's an issue until they start to get bullied. Generally speaking, children can be very insensitive and any child that is different and a stuttering child is very different from a fluent child may get picked on. This will cause the child to avoid speaking situations and he/she will see themselves as outsiders.

Bullying has changed from my time in school, the immergence of mobile phones and the Internet has taken bullying to new dimensions and escalated the severity of bullying so the child cannot even escape the taunts when they are home. Sometimes a child that is bullied will receive malicious emails and the bully may pass the email address on to other children for the vicious campaign to be escalated. Bullying can continue in chat rooms and discussion forums. The child can receive text messages and calls of taunting or even threats.

It is important that parents monitor behavioural patterns if they think a child is being bullied, if a child is spending more time alone in their room, not wanted to go out or has a loss of appetite than you should recognise these as tell tale signs. Stuttering children that are being bullied may be affected to such a degree that their school work is affected as well as their self-esteem; they may also suffer from anxiety, nightmares and paranoia of school and other children. I remember walking in to secondary school with children walking behind me calling me a spastic. What the term spastic has to do with stuttering is still a mystery to me.

Nevertheless, at that time this caused me a huge amount of pain. When I suffered a severe block the laughter of the children would really hurt. I think my English teacher took some sort of sick pleasure in asking me to stand up and read something out, he knew I stuttered, offering no practical advice and letting me get humiliated by my class mates.

As you can imagine I avoided English lessons, a child that is suffering bullying may avoid certain classes. I have also read about some children that have even attempted suicide due to severe bullying.

Parent's role

If you feel as though your child is being bullied then your first step should be to approach your child. Make sure your words and body language portray a supportive, understanding parent.

Bullying has taken on new dimensions as violent crime has increased over the last 20 years, especially when there is easy availability of knives and guns. So asking the child to deal with the bullies is not a wise idea. You should always encourage the child to inform the teacher, form tutor or head of year either via a note in the bully box (if the school has one) or via a letter to the teacher. All schools are obliged by the law to tackle bullying and have polices and procedures in place regarding bullying.

Make sure as you are speaking to your child that you write down the names of the children involved, witnesses, incidents and if you feel as though your child has been physically assaulted, take him/her to a doctor for this to be recorded.

I can imagine myself if I knew my son had been bullied because of his stutter and physically assaulted, it would be hard for me not too lose my temper. However, I would have to remain calm and would recommend to others to do the same. If you lose your temper it will scare your child and not provide a long term solution to the problem but rather a short term fix.

You should arrange a meeting with a class teacher, form tutor or head of year to discuss this issue. The issue may be resolved at this stage by bringing it to the teacher's attention. If your child has been seriously physically assaulted then your first port of call should be to inform the police as the issue has already escalated to a dangerous level. In most cases it will be taunting and persistent bullying.

You may have to write a formal letter to the head teacher and request a meeting with the head teacher and head of governors. At this stage you should bring a GP report if necessary, speech therapist reports and a detailed log of everything you have kept. Make sure that your concerns are addressed and a plan of action is agreed; Keep in regular contact with the head teacher to see if they are making progress.

The most important action you can do is to communicate with your child, building a rapport to make sure that the bullying never happens again. Remember you have to be a friend to the child rather than the traditional parent child relationship that you may have had in your formative years. It may be necessary to change their mobile number and email address.

Keep complimenting the child and make a conscious effort to build up their self-esteem. The worse case scenario isn't the child being bullied as this can be resolved; it's that the bullying will affect their self confidence which will have a knock on effect later in life.

Bullying at the work place is also classed as harassment and is defined as violating someone's personal dignity or creating a degrading or offensive environment. If you are being bullied at work due to your stuttering then you should approach your employer who as a legal obligation to address the complaint, if you feel that the issue is still not being resolved then you can visit your union for advice. Make sure you keep a log of all the incidents that have taken place and if possible record the conversations with an mp3 player.

Being harassed or taunted at work due to your stutter is unacceptable and no one should have to put up with it.

Advice for Parents

The role of the parents is vital in supporting the development of the child's speech and language skills. Parents usually are the first to notice dysfluency and this can cause feelings of being helpless and they will very often adopt the role of a speech therapist. However with very little knowledge about speech therapy they can often worsen the stuttering rather than improving it.

Most parents will approach their family doctor first who will refer them on to a speech and language therapist (SLT). It is important that parents, SLT's and teachers work together to help support a child suffering from stuttering. This chapter will help parents to support and treat a child's stutter and give advice on how they can work effectively with SLT's and teachers.

Initial assessment

After you have been to your doctor you will receive an appointment with an SLT. All children stutter differently and have unique circumstances surrounding their environments. For example a child that is bought up in a bilingual family is at a greater risk of developing a stutter. The SLT will take a detailed assessment of the child's stuttering problem and their speech needs. They will also allow parents to voice their concerns and ask questions regarding what therapy will involve.

The SLT will need to ascertain the severity of the stutter and how it affects the child. Your child's rate of speech and the type of stutter he has will also be analysed.

Some children can be severely affected by the stutter which can cause the child and the parent's psychological distress. The SLT will explore the child's feelings about stuttering. I would also recommend for parents to talk to their child to explore how they feel about the stuttering, this obviously depends on the age of the child.

The SLT may also inquire about your environment, i.e. how many children you have, how much time you spend with your child, the child's hobbies/ dislikes and the child's personality. These psychological factors affect the child's language skills and social life at school.

How you Communicate with your Child

It is important to realise that as parents we did not cause our child to stutter but we can help a child to overcome his stutter. It is essential that parents instil confidence in their child's communication. When at home talk to your child at a slower speech and continue this new talking habit with your spouse. Increase pauses between sentences and pay special attention to listening to the child and maintaining eye contact. Being attentive to your child and listening to them will set a good speech example for your child to follow.

Parent Child Interaction Therapy

Parent-Child Interaction Therapy (PCIT) is focused on improving the quality of the parent-child relationship and changing parent-child interaction patterns. In PCIT, parents are taught specific language skills that they implement within the household.

The therapist may recommend sessions with the child and the parents together. At first the SLT will discuss the structure of the session and encourage you to maintain eye contact, praise the child and interact with the child using slow speech. These will be structured play sessions using toys that the child finds interesting which will help the child to replicate the parents speech patterns.

This exercise should also be done at home for at least 10-15 minutes, 3 times a week. It is important you let your child initiate and organise the play session. The SLT may see you every 2 weeks to monitor your progress.

Different activities can be used depending on your child's age and abilities. For example, younger children are introduced to concepts about "slow and fast" talking using puppets and stories. One programme that can be used is to play out the story of the tortoise and the hare which helps your child to understand that "fast" is not necessarily the "best" way. Parents are closely involved in therapy and will have "homework" tasks to carry out between sessions to ensure continuity.

The SLT will also take time to discuss other parenting issues as appropriate. Being a parent is hard work at times and finding ways of dealing with behaviour such as temper tantrums, difficult bedtimes, poor eating etc which can be causing extra anxiety due to stuttering. Many parents are worried about being too strict with their child in case their stuttering worsens.

Older children will be given lots of help to understand the complexity of stuttering and problem-solving skills to help them to help themselves in a variety of ways.

These parent child interaction sessions will help in improving fluency within the household and will have a positive effect in the child stuttering. However your child may need to develop some fluency tools that will help him when they are stuttering. Your child will need to understand the concepts of:

- Talking Slowly
- Talking Smoothly
- Talking easily without struggling

If the child still struggles after parent child interaction sessions then the SLT will focus on developing the above points and may progress your child on to direct therapy.

Direct Therapy

Some SLT's will recommend you to the Lidcombe Programme. The Lidcombe Programme is a treatment developed specifically for stuttering in children younger than six. However, it is known to be effective also with school-age children. The Lidcombe Program is based on encouraging the child to use smooth speech. When he does then you praise the child by empathising the smoothness of the speech i.e. "wasn't that smooth then", "you didn't get stuck, and that was smooth". An idea would be to give the child a sticker that he could stick on to a talking chart on the kitchen fridge. After so many fluent conversations the child would get a treat such as ice cream.

If the child does stutter then the parents must recognise by emphasizing getting "stuck" or being "bumpy" this is done by saying "you got stuck there" or "lets try that again without the stuck word". It is very important that parents remain positive and supportive of the child. The child needs to enjoy the treatment.

As is the case with any treatment for a childhood speech and language disorder, it will not work if the child does not enjoy it and feels it is not a positive experience. Most important of all in the Lidcombe Programme, care is taken that parental feedback is not constant, intensive or invasive. The emphasis of the Lidcombe programme is for the child to manage their own stutter as the programme is individualised for every family.

Nursery Children

Stuttering usually emerges during the nursery years as the child first begins to have conversations using sentences. Children at this stage tend to have dysfluencies as they have so much to say and they feel as though they need to get it all out at once. So a child may suffer from repetitive or hesitant speech patterns.

The parents and nursery staff will instinctively realise if a child's dysfluency is not normal but is actually a stutter. At this stage it would be wise to have a meeting with the nursery staff. You may wish to have informal conversations with the nursery staff to see if they have noticed his dysfluency. This could be followed by a formal meeting.

It is important to consider risk factors associated with your child developing a stutter as opposed to a child "growing out" of the dysfluency. Factors include, is there is a genetic link to stuttering? Has your child been stuttering for over a year? Does your child have difficulties in language development? If you answer yes to any of these questions then you should visit your doctor and ask for a referral to a SLT.

It is important to find out if your child is aware of his dysfluency. Some children will not be aware of their stuttering until it gets pointed out to them. Others will realise that something is wrong when they are talking which can cause them to flinch or mention it to their parents.

Dysfluency in young children can vary from good weeks to bad weeks. My son's stuttering varies incredibly and sometimes you can forget he has a stutter until he has a few bad weeks which set's alarm bells ringing in my head. There is no real pattern to stuttering at this age so it can be confusing what triggers those bad days.

The child is more likely to struggle with his speech if he is talking about something complicated or if he is put on the spot and asked a direct question.

Don't say the Word for the Child

As parents it's hard to watch your child struggle when talking and a natural reaction is to help your child by completing the word. You may be uncomfortable watching the child but the child may be unaware of any tension and just persevere until they complete the word they have blocked on. As a parent you feel frustrated and have a sense of helplessness but you must avoid finishing the child's word for them as it will affect the child's confidence. In fact it's important that you tell your child to take his time with he gets stuck on a word. This will encourage your child to slow down their speech which in turn will increase their fluency.

It is also important that you treat all your children equally and not favour a stuttering child as this will ensure that the child does not think of himself as different. Also help your other children to realise that they should allow him more time to talk and not to tease him.

Your Speech

Setting a good example about speech patterns will help your child manage their stutter. Pausing for a few seconds before answering your child will set the example that you are organising thoughts. As your child notices how you are answering his question he will replicate your speech patterns over time and develop this skill which will help his fluency.

This thinking time before you talk allows the child to compose their thoughts and slow down their speech pattern.

Also speaking to your child in a calm, slow fashion is essential. Start off by talking in this manner for short periods of time and then extend the periods gradually until it has a beneficial effect on your child's stuttering. Be aware of your body language; make sure it doesn't communicate frustration.

Stuttering can also worsen with longer complicated sentences and when the child has a rapidly growing vocabulary. Television, radio and the Internet are increasing children's vocabulary at a quicker rate. When you speak to your child try and keep the vocabulary and the sentence structure simple.

The child will develop a greater vocabulary as they get older but it important for them to grasp the fluency of some key sounds at this stage.

Taking Turns

If you have more than one child then they may all compete to say something to you. This can cause a stuttering child to suffer a dysfluency as they are trying to rush the words. It is important as parents we encourage the child to raise their hands and take turns to talk. This will allow the child to understand that he has time to talk and there is no rush to complete the sentence. If the child does stutter, keep eye contact, do not say the word for them and show patience.

Primary school

Some children that stutter at primary school start to talk fluently by the time they get to secondary school. However a large percentage of children can continue to stutter. Children at this age can have associated body language when they stutter that will demonstrate frustration such as foot stamping.

A primary school child may be becoming increasingly aware that their speech is different from their friends. He may also make a conscious effort to avoid problem words or sounds. Your child may also avoid situations where he would need to talk such as raising their hands in class to answer questions.

A child may also use fillers such as "err" and "umm" more frequently to break up difficult words into segments. Just like primary nursery school children, primary school children go through bouts of fluency followed by dysfluency. It's not possible to explain to a child of this age about the concept of fear, relaxation techniques and complex intervention techniques. However, we can reduce the frequency in stuttering and provide the child with ways to manage their stutter.

As parents we will become even more anxious as we can envisage the child being teased and his education being affected. Much of the advice given to nursery children, I think is still relevant such as not finishing off sentences, keeping eye contact, encouraging the child to speak and complimenting him when he talks fluently.

What advice should I give my child?
It is a natural reaction to ask your child to breathe more when they are stuttering. However, this can result in build up of tension which can cause the child to stutter. It is better to just listen and be patient at this age.

Don't push him to talk in public but similarly do not assume that he cannot talk in public due to his stutter. Let your child decide if he wants to talk in front of extended family, friends, assembly in school or even school plays and dramas. Some children do not stutter when they are performing in a play. This may be due to them emphasizing words. Also talking or singing in unison can help a child's fluency.

Acknowledgment

If the child is aware that they stutter then you should acknowledge them when they stutter by saying something like; "it was hard to say that wasn't it?" also praise the child "you tried really hard to say that word, well done!"

Try not to talk about his stutter in front of other relatives or friends. Talk to him alone as it will save him from embarrassment.

Working with School Teachers

It is essential that your child's school teacher is aware of his stuttering and the treatment plan you have in place for him.

A simple change to the daily routine like asking the children to raise their hands at register may help to increase fluency as the child is put under pressure of saying his name and stuttering. This tension during register time can be worse if your child has had his fellow class mates laugh at him in the past. Another alternative is that children are given name cards that they can show the teacher at registration. These changes largely depend on the type of teacher your child has and if they are willing to change their daily routines.

A child is also more likely to stutter when reading aloud to the class or to the teacher. This can cause serious distress and can even result in tears or a tantrum. Ask the teacher to read in unison with your child as this is usually very beneficial and encourages fluency. Make sure the teacher reads in a calm slow manner so your child replicates this speech pattern.

You can also mention to the teacher that it is vitally important that we show patience with our body language when the child is suffering a block. Sometimes teachers nod their heads which can be communicated to a child as "hurry up I'm in a rush".

Encourage the teacher to let children take turns when speaking. This practice may already be present in schools but emphasising the importance of it for a stuttering child may be necessary. This can slow down the speech of your child and encourage him to organise his thoughts and to take small pauses before answering questions which will in turn produce more fluent speech.

If your child continues to stutter towards the end of their time at primary school then realistically they will not overcome their stutter easily. You will have to find ways that your child can manage their stutter until they are ready for more intensive therapy. As parents we must make sure that the stutter does not affect the child emotionally or educationally.

Teasing and Bullying

In the early years of primary school the child is more likely to be teased than bullied. Please refer to the bullying chapter for further advice on bullying. I can tell you from personal experiences that being teased in primary school by being laughed at or mimicked can turn a young child's life into misery.

I still remember being teased at primary school and I'm in my 30's now. Other children may giggle when your child stutters; this may not even be malicious and may be due to feeling uncomfortable, this is a natural reaction for children at this age.

Teachers may not be aware of the teasing going on as it may happen during lunch or breaks. It is important that you communicate with your child to find out who was responsible and how they feel. You could approach the school teacher and bring it their attention but I'm a firm believer that a child should be allowed to find their own solutions to their stuttering problems.

If you feel as though you should approach the teacher then make sure a plan of action is agreed upon and the child gets feedback from the teacher that they have spoken to the children responsible. In my opinion and many teachers and SLT's will most probably disagree with me here, I feel that there will always be another child that teases your child. You cannot reprimand the whole school and the child will also get accused of "telling" or if you prefer slang "grassing up". As long as the teasing has not escalated into physical violence then I feel the child should be encouraged to find ways he can deal with children that tease him. It's important that we distinguish between teasing which could be mimicking and name calling and swearing. If the child is being called names or being sworn at then this should always be bought to the attention of the teacher.

Usually the child's closest friends will not tease him, they may ask him out of curiosity why the he talks like that. At this stage it's important for the teacher to teach the whole class about learning to accept the differences in each other. For example we have different colour skin, different colour hair, we eat different foods at home and if someone talks differently then this does not mean he is strange. It just means that we are all unique.

Secondary School

Children at secondary schools go through enormous emotional and physical changes. Puberty affects children in many different ways and it is hard enough dealing with these physical and emotional changes as well as coping with a stutter.

There's pressure to wear the right clothes, with the right labels, and to have the right appearance. Everywhere you look - TV, magazines, shops - children are confronted by advertisements which show you what you should be doing/ wearing/ saying/ buying. Having to cope with all this as well as a stutter can take its toll on the child.

The role of the parent's decreases in the child's everyday life as they form new bonds with friends and the pressures associated with these new relationships. Language skills are also going to be more complicated as they move towards GCSE's or the equivalent qualification in your country for 11 year olds.

How Children Manage their own Stutter

The child's fear of frustration and embarrassment will be peaking at this age and as such they will find ingenious but often counter productive ways in dealing with their stutter. Children may use fillers such as "erm" and "ahhh" more frequently or avoid using certain words altogether. Some children will avoid answering questions at home and in the classroom.

The fear of suffering a block in class may cause some children to be disruptive by swearing or telling jokes to class mates. They are usually relaxed while playing the class joker and tend not to stutter and talk fluently. This can cause the teacher to send the pupil out of class as they are disrupting the others children's education and this will get the child out of talking. This is a short term fix for the child from being ridiculed but the long term educational impact is huge. Often a child may develop a large vocabulary and simply make a conscious effort to avoid certain words so no one would be aware that they have a stutter. This is another short term fix as they cannot continue to avoid words and not use the English language to its fullest for the rest of their education.

Situations

Certain situations will put the child under more pressure. Speaking to the opposite sex can often have the child in knots. They don't want to be laughed at and may avoid it altogether.

If the teenager does speak to the opposite sex they may get hot or sweaty, heart pounding, butterflies in the stomach are also natural as this is how the body responds to strong emotions. The difference with a stuttering teenager is that if they do suffer ridicule due to their stuttering in front of the opposite sex then this can seriously affect their self confidence. This can result in feeling isolated and the worse case scenario is that a child can get depressed and consider self harm.

The teenager will also avoid answering questions in class and the thought of doing an oral examination would be terrifying. The teenager may not only fear the reaction of their fellow students but also the teacher. They don't want to be thought of as being stupid or not as bright as other students. In most cases if you encourage your teenager to speak to the teacher and explain the problem they can work together on the stuttering problem.

As parents it is important we continue to have the same relationship with the secondary school teacher as we had with the nursery and primary school teachers. Some teachers imply that they do not know how to manage a child that stutters so giving a person basic advice like waiting for him to finish the block, not guessing the word, keeping eye contact and speaking in a calm manner will help.

Also changing the way the teacher decides who will read aloud in class may be necessary. You could suggest to the teacher that rather than dominating a person to read out aloud you could ask for volunteers. This will enable the stuttering teenager to choose if he is having a "good day" and is confident about talking or not. Also as discussed earlier reading in unison can help fluency. If the student has great difficulty in answering the question then the teacher should be encouraged to point out what a good answer he gave.

If you encourage the child and praise him in front of his peers it will increase his self confidence.

Sometimes a student may be required to read something aloud for an oral examination. In this case make sure the teacher gives him plenty of warning so that he can practice at home. Ask your child to read to you at home and concentrate on pausing after commas and full stops, also try and get your child to emphasise key words in a sentence. At this stage practical advice from the "let's talk" chapter can be implemented.

Special Consideration

In some cases you may feel that your child cannot emotionally do an English oral examination. In this case you can apply to the examination board for special considerations. This will allow the student to only be assessed on their written work but their certificate will say that. This would be a last resort as this could affect their prospects for further education or work. A better option would be for the SLT and the parents to work together on the English oral examination so the student can overcome he's fear of the exam.

Recap

As a parent you have the support you need with SLT's and teachers to help you to increase your child's fluency. The advice given in this chapter is brief but very concise and can be used throughout your child's educational development. It's important that you use the strategies that you will advocate to teachers yourself at home. As a parent of a child that stutters I know how frustrating it can be to watch your child stutter but now that you have a greater understanding of how to overcome stuttering, you can help your child to speak fluently.

Printed in the United Kingdom
by Lightning Source UK Ltd.
130867UK00001B/172-264/P